Microbiology and Immunology Casebook

Microbiology and Immunology Casebook

James T. Barrett, Ph.D.

Professor Emeritus of Microbiology and Immunology, University of Missouri–Columbia School of Medicine, Columbia, Missouri; Professor of Microbiology, and Deputy Chairman of Pathology/Microbiology, St. George's University, Grenada, West Indies

Little, Brown and Company
Boston New York Toronto London

First Edition

Library of Congress Cataloging-in-Publication Data

Barrett, James T., 1927–
Microbiology and immunology casebook / James T. Barrett
p. cm.
Includes bibliographical references and index.
ISBN 0-316-08132-9
1. Medical microbiology—Case studies. 2. Immunology—Case studies. 3. Medical immunology—Examinations, questions, etc. 4. Immunology—Examinations, questions, etc. I. Title.
[DNLM: 1. Microbiology—examination questions. 2. Microbiology—case studies. 3. Allergy and Immunology—case studies. 4. Allergy and Immunology—examination questions. QW 18.2 B274m 1995]
QR46.B355 1995
616'.01'076—dc20
DNLM/DLC
for Library of Congress 95-13078
CIP

Printed in the United States of America

MV-NY

Editorial: Evan R. Schnittman, Suzanne Jeans
Copyeditor: Debra Corman
Indexer: Alexandra Nickerson
Production Services: Pageworks
Cover Designer: Design Heads
Cover Illustration: Peg Gerrity

Contents

Preface

Nothing pleases a medical student more than a compilation of old examinations except perhaps a review book with 20 to 50 questions per chapter or a computer program containing hundreds of questions. Students sort through such questions by the hour, attempting to acquire the proficiency they need to pass an examination. While it is probably true that old examinations may offer insight about a professor's prejudices and guide the student through those prejudices at examination time, educators are doubtful that old exams, computer quizzes, or review questions are truly effective means of learning.

The move to problem based learning (PBL) presented among its benefits an indoctrination into a learning mode with lifelong applicability based on the origination and resolution of questions developed by the student. Certainly the medical vignettes used in PBL exercises are generally more interesting than a droning lecturer and a lecture outline. But, as with any system of learning, personal assessment of one's knowledge base is useful, and often comforting, when proven satisfactory. The best method for reviewing PBL exercises is by working through more PBL problems, not cramming with old examinations or computer quizzes.

Problem casebooks should offer more than a medical vignette with four or five questions and their appended answers. Rather, such books should cause the student to seek answers to numerous pertinent questions about that case in a true PBL scenario. Even more important, the student's curiosity about related situations should be stimulated to consider more distantly related questions.

These two conditions culminated in the single goal of this book: to provide cases with specific questions and a section of open-ended questions. Each medical vignette is followed by a few unanswered questions closely related to the case. It is important for the student to develop an answer, not simply to memorize the single answer provided. Many a false comfort has arisen from reading an answer and thinking, "Yes, I knew that all right" without fully considering what the answer might be before reading it. Because the student is directly involved in the problem solving scenario, he or she gains the opportunity to formulate new questions more distantly related to the case. When this is accomplished faithfully a broad range of information can be reviewed. Because of the need for knowledge assessment in the PBL framework, this dual approach is recommended for those coming from a PBL background or facing it in licensing examinations. This casebook is designed in part for self-assessment, though it may equally well serve PBL goals in the classroom.

J.T.B.

Acknowledgments

Several cases in this book have been used by my former and current students. I am indebted to them for their criticisms, which I hope reflect their intent to improve these cases.

Very important to me on a practical scale has been the superb assistance provided by my secretaries, Karen Ehlert and Venicia James. They are indeed examples of the computer generation at its highest level of proficiency.

And at Little, Brown and Company, my sincere appreciation to Evan Schnittman for his enthusiastic support of this project; to Tom Manning, a friend of many years; and to Suzanne Jeans.

I

Medical Microbiology

Notice

1 Problem Cases and How to Use Them

The problem cases in this book have been developed for, and in some instances tested with, second-year medical students studying medical microbiology and immunology. These cases span the normal content of such courses. Part I contains problem cases in basic microbiology, pathogenic bacteriology, virology, mycology, and parasitology. Part II is restricted to immunology and is divided into chapters on immunity, immunoassays, immunodeficiency, transplantation immunology, tumor immunology, autoimmunity, and allergy.

These cases can be an effective addition to traditional lecture-based courses. The tendency to reduce "wet labs" in medical school courses has freed the time needed to add problem cases to the so-called standard curriculum. This can now be done without penalty to any lecture component of the course. A less structured but equally valuable approach might employ these problem cases as substitutes for a few lectures. When used in this way, the instructors can usually ensure that the significant facts of the replaced lecture are uncovered during discussion of the problem case. A third alternative is to develop a course exclusively around cases, in which instance a careful selection of these and other cases would be required to present a balanced course. Application of the problem cases in this manner must be within a time framework that allows an intensive analysis of the case and associated conditions.

Student Use of Problem Cases

Developing Your Information Base

Virtually every case in this book represents a potential encounter a physician will have during medical practice. Unlike multidisciplinary problems that are designed as instructional umbrellas for all basic science subjects, these cases are limited to the disciplines of microbiology and immunology. It is doubtful if a multidisciplinary case-based program can develop the depth of information in microbiology and immunology that these discipline-specific problems will encompass. By focusing on a specific unit in the medical curriculum, students can achieve a depth of knowledge that will be very gratifying. More importantly, this information should prove useful not only on a short-term basis (i.e., your current course) but also in the longer view (i.e., in your clinical years). This is especially important for those who are contemplating an infectious disease specialty after graduation.

Too frequently case study texts provide a medical history and follow that with some half-dozen questions, which are then answered in the subsequent pages. In one sense this defeats the primary purpose of the problem case as a learning instrument by implying that there are only those half-dozen important facts to be learned from a case. In the format used for the 112 problem cases in this book, answers are not provided, and you, the student, are expected to determine what you want to learn from the problem case. Questions, usually 10 or fewer, are listed with each case as primers for the most obvious information that should be garnered from the problem case. These questions should be considered only as such, and many additional questions can be posed for each scenario.

These questions are thus easily separated into distinct levels. The first-level questions can be described as core questions that will apply to virtually every case. The following is a partial list of what may be considered as core questions for Part I:

1. What is the probable microbiologic etiology of the infection?
2. What are the major characteristics of that agent?
3. What other agents may cause this type of disease?
4. What other agents resemble the probable pathogen?
5. What are the major virulence properties of the suspected pathogen?
6. How does one establish the microbiologic diagnosis of this case?
7. What serologic tests are available to assist in the laboratory diagnosis? What are the expected results of these tests?
8. Is the disease preventable by immunization?
9. What means other than immunization are important in the control of the disease?
10. How is the disease acquired or spread?
11. What is the preferred antibiotic or other treatment of the disease?

It is unlikely that your instructor will be satisfied by answers to such core questions alone. Your second-level questions should consider fundamental details related to the agent and the case. You will need, via questions, to demonstrate a curiosity about the nature of the vaccine (is it an attenuated or recombinant vaccine?), the mode of action of certain related toxins, the chemical characteristics and genetic origin of these toxins, the role of plasmids in antibiotic resistance, and so on, as these relate to the case.

It is possible that your professors will be totally satisfied by answers to these second-level questions, but if not, you will be expected to move into even more distant, third-level considerations. If you have an obvious case of bacterial pneumonia, after you consider first- and second-level questions about bacterial pneumonia, you should progress to these same kinds of questions about pneumonia caused by fungi, viruses, and animal parasites. If your third-set questions first consider viral pneumonia due to the influenza virus, you may eventually pose questions such as the following:

1. What are the structural components of this virus?

2. What are the implications of the fact that this is a negative-stranded, segmented RNA virus?
3. What are antigenic drift and antigenic shift from the viewpoint of viral genetics and replication?
4. Is this an enveloped or naked virus?
5. Is chemotherapy of influenza or any viral pneumonia possible?

The list would obviously continue through other agents of pneumonia, but remember that these questions about influenza arose from an initial consideration of a case of bacterial pneumonia. You will be expected to "free think" your way through the broad field of the pneumonias, the diarrheas, the sexually transmitted diseases, and so on, when confronted with a single case within any one of these subject areas. Although practically all cases are in themselves rather direct, you and your instructor can make them as broad and as informative as you wish by natural progressions into related areas.

The usual medical case book adds to each case or section a handful of references from which the case was developed or which solve one or two aspects of the case. Here again, this book differs. In this volume, each chapter has an introductory section that contains data in a descriptive format, frequently condensed into tables, that are useful in solving problem cases in that chapter. For this same reason, the Information Sources are broader in scope than those traditionally found in case books. A major goal in problem-based learning is not simply to solve the problem case but to have or develop resources that will enable you to solve these and similar cases. Another feature seldom found in other case history books is the Key Words and Phrases list. It will be noted that the key words and phrases (which often include abbreviations as well) are not limited to the individual cases in the chapter, again directing attention to the general area of the chapter's focus rather than to a few limited cases. Further emphasis to the expansive concept in the use of these problem cases is seen in the Review Questions, many of which relate to situations not included in the chapter but refer to additional, similar cases.

Review for Examinations

Regardless of the curriculum of your medical school, problem-solving cases will be useful in your review preparation for examinations. Whether you are in a classic or problem-based curriculum, problem-based examinations are in your future. The National Board of Medical Examiners has developed the new licensing examination on the premise that problems are what physicians meet in actual practice and that licensing examinations should reflect this. Clearly, past experience in analyzing case history problems will provide an advantage in this national examination.

In classic, lecture-based curricula, where groups of microorganisms are considered one-by-one, there eventually becomes a need to relate these organisms to shared organ systems, common diagnostic procedures, common problems in treatment, and so on. Practicing physicians do not examine a patient considering first whether this is a staphylococcal or streptococcal pneumonia, for example. They first try to identify the disease as a pneumonia by seeking its historical clues and by identifying its symptoms and then consider its etiology as it will affect prognosis and treatment. As you ponder these cases, you will be able to identify the key problem without much trouble. The historical clues and presenting symptoms are often classic in their description and are intended to lead you quickly to the microbiologic or immunologic basis of the case. Then you must consider the potential etiology of the case—bacterial, viral, fungal, or parasitic or, in Part II, as an allergy, autoimmune disease, and so on. As you do this, you will be reviewing your lectures from a different viewpoint, and an alternative perspective is an important reinforcement aid to learning and should prepare you well for your examinations.

Case Presentations

In the clinical years of medical school, students are required to present cases to their peers and instructors. The implementation of problem-based exercises in the basic science years of medical school has now introduced student case presentations into this part of the curriculum as well. Students may now be required to present assigned cases that they will describe to their classmates. A logical organization of these presentations will smooth the flow of the data into an intelligible pattern that will facilitate an accurate interpretation of the case. Although variations in the organization of your presentation may be required for certain cases, the following sequence has been used for most problem cases in Part I of this book and is suggested as a guide. A slightly modified approach to the problem cases in Part II will be required.

1. A short, one-sentence description of the patient.

   Example: The patient is a 35-year-old white female in obvious pain.

2. A statement of the chief complaint and its immediate history.

   Example: She had a sudden onset of an explosive diarrhea and lower abdominal pain this morning before contacting her family physician. She complained of a fever and chills.

3. A past medical history that includes only medical situations that impinge on the present illness should be included. A case of scarlet fever 20 years in the past would have no relevance to a current case of diarrhea.

   Example: The patient has had no previous significant abdominal or intestinal complaints.

4. Related family medical history. Current household infections or circumstances that could have contributed to the illness should be included.

   Example: The patient's two children had a mild case of diarrhea earlier this week.

5. Important social data. Factors such as alcoholism, drug abuse, sexual preference or behavior, and travel should be included if they have a bearing on the illness.

Example: The patient's family returned from a vacation in Thailand 2 weeks ago.

6. Associated medical system history. The history of disease or injury to other organ systems that might influence the current situation.

   Example: The patient has no history of abdominal or intestinal disease in the recent past.

7. Pertinent physical findings and vital signs. Typically the patient's body temperature, pulse, respiration rate, and blood pressure are recorded. Other data would be collected—ophthalmologic or neurologic, for example—if pertinent to the case.

   Example: A distended abdomen, odorous flatulence, and gaseous diarrhea were noted. Other organ systems appear normal.

8. Differential diagnosis. A listing or consideration of the possible diseases is established.

   Example: Infectious diarrhea is the probable diagnosis.

9. Laboratory tests and results. Important and even trivial data are often included here. It is sometimes as important to include normal data as data that are more directly related to the case. Many patients in the senior age group will often have two or more concurrent medical conditions or will develop them. A full listing of blood values, urinalysis data, and so on may lead to an identification of these diseases early in their development. For a simple case of diarrhea, possibly only the microbiology laboratory report would be cited.

   Example: No bacterial pathogens were recovered from stool, urine, or blood cultures. Examination for ova and parasites recovered large numbers of *Giardia lamblia* cysts.

10. Confirmed diagnosis. Based on laboratory data and harmonious clinical data, the diagnosis should be confirmed. The reasons why should be clearly stated.

    Example: In the absence of other intestinal pathogens and the presence of *G. lamblia*, the diagnosis is established as diarrhea due to *G. lamblia*. [The difficulty in establishing this diagnosis even in the presence of numerous cysts in the feces should be discussed.]

11. Therapy. Therapeutic options and considerations that led to the final selection should be stated.

    Example: Treatment of giardiasis is controversial. Quinacrine, metronidazole, and nitrofurantoin have all been used in the past. Nitrofurantoin was prescribed at 8 mg/kg/day for 10 days.

12. Current status or outcome. In-house cases require a report of their current status. Discharged patients who need follow-up examinations also require a current status report. If the patient is well, a statement of the outcome is adequate but may not be precisely known.

Example: The patient responded to a telephone interview that she had no further diarrhea 3 days into treatment. The patient has not been recontacted.

Instructor Use of Problem Cases

The movement toward the use of problem-based exercises has already permeated the minds of medical educators, if not their curricula. Whether case studies will soon dominate these curricula is being determined at this time as faculties vote pro or con on this issue. But in a sense this is a nonissue, since problems have always been a part of medical education—in the form of patients in the clinical years and as laboratory unknowns or paper cases in the basic science years. Obviously the ability to solve problems is the key to success in the real world of medical practice.

Undoubtedly many instructors have or will themselves develop a set of their own problem cases. Not only is this time-consuming, but also, as these problems are used in successive years, there is a temptation for students to seek out an upperclassman for answers or precise directions on how to "solve" the problem. This book presents 112 medical vignettes that span the major areas of microbiology and immunology. In a 16-week semester, instructors can select 16, 32, or some other number of cases that suits their schedules. It is realistic to assume that from 112 cases instructors could select one group of cases this year and a completely different set for each of the next 3 years. Alternatively, if problem solving is the dominant component of the course, instructors could use a majority of the cases in a single year.

As mentioned earlier, different instructors will utilize these cases for separate purposes. One avenue is to use them as complete substitutes for lectures. Another approach is to add them to the wet lab as laboratory conferences with the intention to expand or reemphasize aspects of the organisms being examined in the laboratory or lectures at that time. A third possibility is to use them as supplements or replacements in a lecture program of reduced scope.

For use in the classroom, the following format has proved useful. The problem case is assigned to a small group of students by an instructor. The vignette is read, and the students begin to pose and answer questions as a group project based on previous knowledge, however limited that may be. After unanswerable questions are encountered and new questions are created by members of the group, the group disperses to resolve these situations. The group reconvenes subsequently, usually a day or two later, to discuss their answers and share information sources. At this time, doubts and new, more sophisticated questions arise, causing the group to disperse again. A subsequent meeting is held to resolve these further uncertainties. Within this pattern, potentially one or two cases per week could be completed, again depending on the emphasis of problems in that particular course. Even within this projected schedule, advanced details of microbial structure, mechanisms of pathogenesis, genetics of toxin production and antibiotic resistance, vaccine status, basis of immunity, genetics of immunodeficiency conditions, and other vital topics can be discussed.

Chapter assignments for some of these cases have been arbitrary. For example, in

Part I, is brucellosis a food-borne disease or a zoonosis? Is Q fever an airborne disease or a zoonosis? Is chickenpox an airborne disease or a skin and wound infection? On a few occasions, two scenarios of a single condition, placed in different chapters, have been developed to meet this epidemiologic dilemma. The cases in the last chapter of Part I have not been categorized and could be used as a review segment at the end of the course or for self-review.

Information Sources

To create a complete listing of all medical microbiology and immunology texts and review sources useful to medical students is a difficult, if not an impossible, task and hardly necessary. Students are generally aware of the available reference sources, and if not, this listing will guide them to some standard texts used in the United States.

Most medical school libraries will have access through our electronic world to many useful information banks, and medical students obviously need to avail themselves of these facilities.

Part I—Medical Microbiology

Anderson, R.M., and May, R.M.: Infectious diseases of humans, Oxford University Press, 1991, Oxford.

Ballows, A., et al., editors: Manual of clinical microbiology, American Society of Microbiology, 1991, Washington, D.C.

Baron, S., editor: Medical microbiology, edition 3, Churchill Livingstone, 1991, New York.

Belshe, R.B., editor: Textbook of human virology, PSG Publishing Co., 1984.

Bogitsh, B.J., and Cheng, T.C.: Human parasitology, W.B. Saunders Co., 1990, Philadelphia.

Boyd, R.F., and Hoerl, B.G.: Basic medical microbiology, edition 4, Little, Brown, and Co., 1991, Boston.

Braude, A.I., editor: Infectious diseases and medical microbiology, W.B. Saunders Co., 1986, Philadelphia.

Brown, H.W., and Neva, F.A.: Basic clinical parasitology, edition 5, Appleton-Century-Crofts, 1983, Norwalk, CT.

Cook, G.C.: Parasitic disease in clinical practice, Springer-Verlag, 1990, New York.

Davis, B.D., et al., editors: Microbiology, edition 4, J.B. Lippincott Co., 1990, Philadelphia.

Evans, A.S., editor: Viral infections of humans: epidemiology and control, edition 3, Plenum Press, 1989, New York.

Evans, A.S., and Brachman, P.S., editors: Bacterial infections of humans: epidemiology and control, edition 2, Plenum Medical Book Company, 1991, New York.

Evans, E.G.V., and Richardson, M.D.: Medical mycology: a practical approach, Oxford University Press, 1989, Oxford.

Fields, B.N., and Knipe, D.M., editors: Virology, edition 2, Raven Press, 1990, New York.

Freeman, B., et al., editors: Burrow's textbook of microbiology, edition 21, W.B. Saunders Co., 1988, Philadelphia.

Garcia, L.S., and Bruckner, D.A., editors: Diagnostic medical parasitology, ASM Press, 1993, Herndon, VA.

Hoeprich, P.D., and Jordan, M.C., editors: Infectious diseases, edition 4, J.B. Lippincott Co., 1989, Philadelphia.

Isenberg, H.D., editor: Clinical microbiology procedures handbook, ASM Press, 1992, Herndon, VA.

Joklik, W.K., et al., editors: Zinsser Microbiology, edition 20, Appleton and Lange, 1992, Norwalk, CT.

Laroner, D.H.: Medically important fungi, ASM Press, 1993, Herndon, VA.

Mandell, G.L., Douglas, R.G., Jr., and Bennett, J.E., editors: Principles and practice of infectious diseases, edition 3, Churchill Livingstone, 1990, New York.

Markell, E.J., and Voge, M.: Medical parasitology, edition 6, W.B. Saunders Co., 1986, Philadelphia.

Mims, C.A., et al., editors: Medical microbiology, Mosby Europe Limited, 1993, London.

Murray, P.R., et al.: Medical microbiology, edition 2, C.V. Mosby Co., 1994, St. Louis.

Parker, M.T., and Duerden, B.I., editors: Topley and Wilson's Principles of bacteriology, virology, and immunity, Edward Arnold, 1990, Sevenoaks, England.

Persing, D.H., et al., editors: Diagnostic molecular microbiology, ASM Press, 1993, Herndon, VA.

Rippon, J.W.: Medical mycology: the pathogenic fungi and the pathogenic actinomycetes, edition 3, W.B. Saunders Co., 1988, Philadelphia.

Schaechter, M., Medoff, G., and Eisenstein, B.I., editors: Mechanisms of microbial disease, edition 2, Williams & Wilkins, 1993, Baltimore.

Sherris, J.C., editor: Medical microbiology, edition 3, Elsevier Science Pub., 1994, New York.

Shulman, S.T., Phair, J.P., and Sommers, H.M.: The biologic and clinical basis of infectious diseases, edition 4, W.B. Saunders Co., 1991, Philadelphia.

Volk, W.A., et al.: Essentials of medical microbiology, edition 3, J.B. Lippincott Co., 1986, Philadelphia.

White, D.O., and Fenner, F.: Medical virology, edition 3, Academic Press, Inc., 1986, Orlando.

Wiedbrauk, D.L., and Johnston, S.L.G.: Manual of clinical virology, ASM Press, 1993, Herndon, VA.

Wilson, M.E.: A world guide to infections: diseases, distribution, diagnosis, Oxford University Press, 1991, Oxford.

Part II—Medical Immunology

Abbas, A.K., Lichtman, A.H., and Pober, J.S.: Cellular and molecular immunology, edition 2, W.B. Saunders Co., 1994, Philadelphia.

Barrett, J.T.: Medical immunology, text and review, F.A. Davis Co., 1991, Philadelphia.

Benjamini, E., and Leskowitz, S.: Immunology: a short course, edition 2, John Wiley and Sons, 1991, New York.

Bona, C.A., and Bonilla, F.A.: Immunology for medical students, Harwood Academic Publishers, 1990, New York.

Graziano, F.M., and Lemanske, R.F., Jr.: Clinical immunology, Williams & Wilkins, 1988, Baltimore.

Lachmann, P.J., et al., editors: Clinical aspects of immunology, edition 5, Blackwell Scientific Publications, Inc., 1993, Oxford.

Langman, R.E.: The immune system, Academic Press, Inc., 1989, San Diego.

Paul, W.E., editor: Fundamental immunology, edition 3, Raven Press, Inc., 1993, New York.

Roitt, I.: Essential immunology, edition 7, Blackwell Scientific Publications, Inc., 1991, Oxford.

Roitt, I., Brostoff, J., and Male, D.: Immunology, edition 3, J.B. Lippincott Co., 1993, Philadelphia.

Roitt, I.M., and Deeves, P.J., editors: Encyclopedia of immunology, 3 volumes, Academic Press, Inc., 1992, San Diego.

Rosen, F.S., Steiner, L.A., and Unanue, E.R., editors: Dictionary of immunology, Stockton Press, 1988, New York.

Stites, D.P., and Terr, A.I., editors: Basic and clinical immunology, edition 8, Appleton and Lange, 1994, East Norwalk, CT.

Virella, G., et al.: Introduction to medical immunology, edition 3, Marcel Dekker, Inc., 1992, New York.

Widmann, F.K.: An introduction to clinical immunology, F.A. Davis Co., 1989, Philadelphia.

2 Basic Microbiology

The problems in this chapter are concentrated in the area of laboratory methods used in the diagnosis of infectious disease. Problems concerned with the cultivation of bacteria, antibiotic resistance, and bacterial genetics are included, but cases built on virologic methods and serologic diagnosis have been excluded. A separate section of problems in immunology contains the latter.

Unlike later chapters, which provide tabular information and references useful in the approach to the cases, only a few references are listed here. These refer almost exclusively to laboratory procedures in microbiology. Background information on electrophoresis, DNA hybridization, restriction endonucleases, and so on is available in standard texts in biochemistry, genetics, and even general biology. Because the subject matter of the cases in this chapter is less focused than in later chapters, no attempt to tabulate this material has been made.

The breadth of material contained in this chapter has also complicated the preparation of the Key Words and Phrases listing. Again, much of the essential vocabulary has already appeared in courses in biochemistry—50S ribosomal unit, folic acid synthetic pathway, restriction fragment length polymorphism, and Northern blot are examples. Rather than repeat terms with which students are already acquainted, the listing in this chapter is limited to terms more directly microbiologic in their origin or use.

Key Words and Phrases

These are but a few of the key words and phrases you should be able to define and explain when you have completed your study of this chapter.

ANTIBIOTICS

Antibiogram

Antibiotic tolerance

Beta lactamase

Beta-lactamase inhibitor

Broad spectrum

Detoxifying enzyme

Kirby-Bauer test

Minimal bactericidal concentration (MBC)

Minimal inhibitory concentration (MIC)

Narrow spectrum

Peptidoglycan synthetic pathway

Resistance transfer factor (RTF)

BACTERIAL GROWTH

Aerobe

Alpha hemolysis

Anaerobe

Bactericidal

Bacteriostatic
Beta hemolysis
Candle jar
Differential medium
Enrichment medium
Facultative
Gamma hemolysis
Microaerophilic
Selective medium
Transport medium

BACTERIAL GENETICS

Bacteriophage typing
Conjugation
F^+
F^-
F'
Hfr
Insertion sequence
Lysogenic conversion
Polymerase chain reaction
Plasmid profile
RFLP
Transduction
Transfection
Transformation
Transposon

Information Sources

Balows, A., et al., editors: Manual of clinical microbiology, edition 5, ASM Press, 1991, Herndon, VA.

Barrow, G.I., and Feltham, R.K.A., editors: Cowan and Steel's Manual for the identification of medical bacteria, edition 3, Cambridge University Press, 1993, Cambridge, England.

Isenberg, H.D., editor: Clinical microbiology procedures, ASM Press, 1992, Herndon, VA.

Klegler, B., et al.: Rapid methods in clinical microbiology, Plenum Press, 1989, New York.

Koneman, E.W., et al.: Color atlas and textbook of diagnostic microbiology, edition 3, J.B. Lippincott Co., 1988, Philadelphia.

Lorian, V., editor: Antibiotics in laboratory medicine, edition 3, Williams & Wilkins, 1991, Baltimore.

Persing, D.H., et al., editors: Diagnostic molecular microbiology, ASM Press, 1993, Herndon, VA.

Washington, J.A. II, editor: Laboratory procedures in clinical microbiology, edition 2, Springer-Verlag, 1985, New York.

Case 1 The Missing Agent

Kim was a recently graduated medical technician who gladly accepted the extra weekend shift. The addition to her paycheck would go a long way toward furnishing her new apartment.

Kim was puzzled by specimen 4395-92. This was a specimen taken from a draining abdominal abscess that she received Saturday evening. The Gram stain revealed the presence of long, slender, pleomorphic, gram-negative bacilli mixed with some more typically formed, shorter bacilli with the same staining reaction. A few gram-positive cocci were also present. When she couldn't find her laboratory procedures notebook, Kim decided to plate the specimen on blood agar and incubate it at 37°C in a candle jar.

Early Sunday morning, when she examined the plate, some very tiny colonies were observed, but Kim decided to wait until Monday when the colonies would be large enough to manipulate before attempting to identify them. On Monday morning, two different colony types were seen. One consisted of gram-positive cocci, later determined to be in the genus *Staphylococcus*. The other colony type had a zone of beta hemolysis around colorless, transparent colonies and was later determined by the IMViC test to be *Escherichia coli*. The *E. coli* cells were short, plump, gram-negative rods. Kim reported these results to her supervisor and commented that the specimen consisted of normal flora.

Questions

1. What is the IMViC test?
2. What is the biochemical basis of each component of the test?
3. Are the media used in the IMViC test selective, differential, or neither?
4. Doesn't hemolysis on a blood agar plate indicate that the isolate is pathogenic?
5. Describe alpha, beta, and gamma hemolysis.
6. Distinguish between an alpha hemolysin and alpha hemolysis or a beta hemolysin and beta hemolysis.
7. What colonial characteristics are useful in the presumptive identification of bacteria?
8. What possibilities explain the failure of Kim to recover slender, pleomorphic, gram-negative bacilli in the cultures?
9. Is blood agar a selective or differential medium?
10. Does a candle jar produce 5% carbon dioxide and anaerobic conditions?
11. What characteristics are used to identify bacteria in the genus *Staphylococcus*?
12. Should Kim have used some type of enrichment medium to isolate the slender, pleomorphic, gram-negative bacillus?

Student Questions

Case 2 The Grade School Demonstration

The students in the sixth grade biology class at Ulysses S. Grant Elementary School had to select a research project for demonstration to the rest of the class. Beth's father was a microbiologist, and he showed her how to do an antibiotic disk sensitivity assay with *Staphylococcus aureus*. Beth determined that the zone of growth inhibition for six common antimicrobial agents was as indicated:

Antimicrobial	**Diameter (mm)**
Penicillin G, 10 U	19
Methicillin, 1 μg	17
Tetracycline, 30 μg	17
Erythromycin, 15 μg	9
Vancomycin, 30 μg	17
Sulfamethoxazole-trimethoprim	7

Beth made several conclusions on her own and then asked her father several questions.

Beth's Conclusions to Be Discussed

1. Since the zone around penicillin is the largest, it is the best antibiotic.
2. All the antibiotics killed the bacteria in areas near the disks.
3. Agents with the same sized zones of inhibition would be equally effective in vivo.
4. Agents with the same sized zones of inhibition kill staphylococci by the same mechanism.
5. Since all the agents inhibited bacterial growth, they are antibiotics.

Questions

1. What are the means by which the antimicrobial agents listed above inhibit the growth of bacteria?
2. Why don't antimicrobials kill human cells? Or do they?
3. Is the disk diffusion method the most accurate means of determining bacterial sensitivity to an antimicrobial?
4. What features determine the size of the zone of inhibition around a disk?
5. Are any of the agents tested also useful against viruses or fungi? Why or why not?
6. Do antimicrobial agents work well in pairs (combination therapy) better than either one alone?
7. Do the antimicrobials always kill the sensitive bacteria?
8. How do bacteria become resistant to antibiotics? Give examples.
9. How is the Kirby-Bauer technique related to the in vivo effectiveness of an antibiotic?

10. What are second-, third-, or later generations of the penicillins and cephalosporins?
11. Which of the antimicrobials Beth tested would be effective in vivo?

Student Questions

Case 3 You Are So Sensitive

Four infants in the newborn nursery of the medical center had staphylococcal infections. Coagulase-positive staphylococci were isolated from all four infants—two with circumcision infections and two with infections of the umbilical stump.

The source of these infections was as yet unknown, but being well aware of the danger of these infections, Dr. Goldstein, Chief of the Hospital Infection Control team, ordered all personnel in the nursery unit to be cultured for carriage of coagulase-positive staphylococci. Several persons had other potentially pathogenic bacteria as part of their normal flora, but only two nurses, Mary C. and Janet S., had the target organism. Through disk diffusion tests by the Kirby-Bauer method, all six staphylococci (four from the infants and two from the nurses) were determined to be resistant to penicillin, erythromycin, and tetracycline. The MIC and the MBC of all six strains were identical.

Questions

1. What is the Kirby-Bauer method?
2. What is the meaning of MIC?
3. How is the MIC determined?
4. What is the meaning of MBC?
5. How is MBC determined?
6. Are the MIC and MBC of an antibiotic ever the same or nearly the same? Why?
7. Would the antibiotic methicillin be useful in treating the sick infants or adults? Why or why not?
8. What are the metabolic targets of penicillin and methicillin?

9. What are penicillin binding proteins?
10. What is the activity of beta lactamase?
11. How are beta-lactamase inhibitors used therapeutically?
12. Which of the three antibiotics is considered to have a narrow spectrum? a broad spectrum?
13. What is the significance of coagulase activity in staphylococci?

Student Questions

Case 4 The Newborn Nursery—Scene 2

Dr. Goldstein decided, after the experience of Case 3, that routine monitoring of the entire staff of the newborn nursery was needed. Since many hospital isolates of staphylococci are resistant to antibiotics, Dr. Goldstein decided to phage type all the staphylococcal isolates. Accordingly, 23 staff members (6 physicians, 8 nurses, 6 assistants, and 3 cleaning and maintenance persons) were cultured by nasopharyngeal swabs. The swabs were placed in transport media and shipped to the State Health Laboratory, where stocks of typing bacteriophage were available.

Although none of the 12 babies in the nursery was ill, swabs were also collected and submitted for analysis from all the infants.

The State Health Laboratory was involved in their own study of the oropharyngeal flora of hospital workers and proceeded to isolate several potentially pathogenic cocci from the specimens, including those of the infants. The following report was sent to Dr. Goldstein:

Isolates from 23 Staff Members		**Isolates from 12 Infants**
Staphylococcus aureus	8	2
Streptococcus pyogenes	1	0
Streptococcus pneumoniae	2	0
Alpha-hemolytic streptococci	23	9
Neisseria meningitidis	3	0

Bacteriophage typing of *S. aureus* isolates

From Staff		From Infants	
Robert B.; M.D.	71	Albert W.	83, 84, 88
Wayne O'D.; M.D.	71/88	Mary S.	83, 84, 88
Jane T.; R.N.	83, 84, 88		
Betty P.; R.N.	55, 71		
Carol E.; R.N.	55, 71		
Ann R.; R.N.	71		
Martha N.; maid	Nontypeable		
Patty D.; maid	71/88		

Questions

1. Are the carrier rates of the cocci within the normal ranges for both the adults and infants?
2. How does the season of the year affect carrier rates?
3. Since *S. aureus* is a pathogen, shouldn't the infants be ill?
4. Assuming that one of the staff members was culture positive for *S. aureus*, *S. pneumoniae*, and *N. meningitidis*, how can that person be well?
5. The State Health Laboratory reported that they used chocolate agar to isolate *N. meningitidis*. How is chocolate agar prepared?
6. How is bacteriophage typing performed?
7. Are phage types an index of bacterial virulence for staphylococci?
8. For what other organisms is phage typing valuable in epidemiologic studies?
9. How many phage types (strains of *S. aureus*) are represented among the staff members?
10. Could there be more than one staff member donor of *S. aureus* to the two infants?
11. Do bacteriophage cause lysogenic conversion to toxin formation in bacteria?
12. Does transduction ever transfer virulence properties between bacteria?

Student Questions

Case 5 Let's Get That in Profile

The first thought Ken Camp had on viewing his plates was that this was going to be pretty embarrassing.

The problem surfaced when four of the last six cardiac bypass patients developed septicemia due to *Staphylococcus epidermidis*. The Hospital Infection Control Committee immediately began a search to identify the source of the infections. *Staphylococcus epidermidis* was isolated from eight people in the cardiac surgery team and four in the cardiac intensive care unit (CICU). Five people in the surgical team and six in the CICU were not colonized. All 12 of the isolates appeared identical based on the usual biotyping panel of sugar fermentations, enzyme assays, and antibiogram. It was then that Ken suggested doing either a bacteriophage or plasmid profile. Since he didn't have a set of typing phage or wish to notify the State Health Laboratory of the problem as yet, he chose plasmid profiling.

DNA was extracted from the four patient isolates, the eight members of the cardiac surgery staff, and the four people from the CICU and examined by gel electrophoresis.

Questions

1. How does one identify bacterial chromosomal DNA as different from plasmid DNA?
2. Is it possible to have more than one DNA band from plasmid DNA? Describe conjugative and non-conjugative plasmids.
3. Would you expect all the bypass parients to have identical plasmid profiles.?
4. How would you identify that the CICU staff have plasmid profiles identical to that of the patients?
5. What virulence properties are associated with staphylococcal plasmids and plasmids of other bacteria?
6. Do plasmid types of staphylococci isolated from patients differ from year to year or from one disease to another?
7. Do certain phage types associate with certain plasmid types?
8. How does the laboratory determine more exactly that plasmids of the same size are identical?
9. Is plasmid typing more exact than phage typing?
10. What other pathogenic bacteria are subject to exact identification via plasmid profiling?
11. Is a plasmid a transposon?
12. Explain conjugation as a means of transfer of F^+, F', and Hfr plasmids.

Student Questions

Case 6 Direct RFLP

Tom F. was a new technician in the clinical microbiology laboratory. His speciality was parasitology and mycology, subjects that several of his coworkers seemed to dislike. As part of Tom's employment, he was given the liberty to test some new diagnostic procedures to prepare a report for the national convention.

Tom was especially interested in three successful cultivations of *Acanthamoeba* from specimens supplied by the Ophthalmology Division. The ophthalmologists were concerned about cases of corneal keratitis appearing in contact lens users. In their search for an infectious etiology, they had sent specimens to Tom on a regular basis. As soon as he had perfected his culture technique with known strains of *Acanthamoeba*, Tom isolated the amoeba on three occasions. To identify the organism more precisely, he extracted and precipitated DNA from all three isolates. He subsequently digested the preparations with RNase prior to exposing each to restriction enzyme cleavage by endonucleases *Eco*RI, *Bam*HI, and *Pst*I. A culture of a known pathogenic strain and a nonpathogenic strain were treated in an identical fashion. After agarose gel electrophoresis, the DNA bands were developed.

Questions

1. How is DNA from the clinical isolates proven to be identical on the basis of DNA fragment analysis?
2. Is the DNA profile of a clinical isolate always identical to that of a pathogenic strain?
3. What are obvious problems in the analysis of RFLP profiles?
4. How would direct DNA probing simplify this procedure?
5. What are the sources and linkage specificity of *Eco*RI, *Bam*HI, and *Pst*I?
6. Is DNA cleavage by three endonucleases sufficient to determine that two samples are identical?
7. What was the purpose of digesting the RNA with ribonuclease?
8. Can one determine from electrophoresis of DNA fragments if the amoebae contain plasmids?
9. What is the definition of transfection? Are amoebae susceptible to transfection?
10. What extrachromosomal forms of DNA have been found in amoebae?

Student Questions

Case 7 Polymerase Chain Reaction

Dr. Ralstedt was perplexed. This was the third report this month from the histology laboratory with identical descriptions of frozen-section biopsies of lymph nodes taken from AIDS patients. Each report described the expected effects of AIDS on lymph node structure and lymphocyte counts, but each also contained a description of tiny bacillus-like cells present in the tissue specimens. Special stains were needed to detect these organisms, which were also seen in liver biopsies from these same patients.

Dr. Ralstedt checked his microbiology laboratory computer printouts one more time. None of the cultures of lymph nodes from these patients had ever yielded bacteria. It certainly wasn't a fault of his technicians; his laboratory had the highest ranking in the state by the accrediting board. Dr. Ralstedt decided to call Dr. Forrest in the DNA Research Unit.

After Dr. Forrest heard Dr. Ralstedt's description of the situation with these three patients, he proposed that they run a polymerase chain reaction (PCR) on some of the DNA extracted from the patient's lymph node. Dr. Forrest explained that DNA from the lymph nodes could be amplified by the PCR technique and that several different primers could be used. Synthetic DNA primers with sequences copied from ribosomal RNA of eukaryotes were chosen. Dr. Forrest stated that he could begin the PCR run as soon as he received frozen lymph node tissue from a control.

The next week Dr. Forrest asked Dr. Ralstedt to stop by the DNA laboratory to see the results. He explained to Dr. Ralstedt that they had expanded the DNA from the samples by the PCR method. These DNA samples were cut with endonucleases and inserted into a plasmid that was placed in a strain of *Escherichia coli*. The bacteria were then grown in culture to expand the DNA. The plasmid DNA was extracted from the bacteria and separated from chromosomal DNA by gel electrophoresis. The eluted plasmid DNA was sequenced, and this sequence was searched in a computer file of DNA gene sequences. This DNA had a 93% sequence agreement with the DNA of *Bacillus nonexistencis* and was thus identified as a new pathogen of AIDS patients.

Questions

1. Explain the PCR technique.
2. How is the PCR DNA product inserted into a plasmid?
3. What is the restriction of a restriction endonuclease?
4. What is blunt-end cleavage by restriction endonucleases?
5. What is sticky-end cleavage by restriction endonucleases?
6. How does one select primers for PCR expansion of DNA?
7. How could one use PCR in the identification of RNA viruses?
8. What pathogenic organisms are most ideally identified by the PCR technique?
9. What is the time required for PCR analysis compared to the isolation of pathogenic bacteria, viruses, and so forth?
10. How could PCR and RFLP be combined for the identification of DNA? What advantages would this offer over PCR alone?
11. Distinguish between transfection and transformation.

Student Questions

Case 8 DNA Probe

Tom F. always opened his mail with the wastebasket nearby. He was expecting the usual announcements of meetings, a few book ads, and maybe a journal or newsletter. He wasn't disappointed and quickly recycled the bulk of the mail, but the newsletter was more interesting. An ad on page 2 indicated that Development Nucleic Associates had developed a new DNA probe specific for *Acanthamoeba* (see Case 6). Tom wrote to the company, informed them of his restriction fragment length polymorphism study, and requested a trial sample of the new probe.

When the probe kit arrived, Ken followed the directions for extracting DNA from his three clinical isolates and the known virulent and avirulent strains of *Acanthamoeba* and subjected all the samples to gel electrophoresis. Thereafter, he applied the probe and analyzed the results.

Questions

1. Could several bands "light up" with a probe specific for a virulent strain or only one band?
2. What conclusions would prove the probe is specific for pathogenic *Acanthamoeba*?
3. How could this test be applied to the diagnosis of a latent infection with a DNA virus?
4. Could RNA in the amoebas be hybridizing with the DNA probe? How could this be controlled?
5. What is the difference between Northern, Southern, and Western blotting?
6. What DNA probes are now available for pathogenic microorganisms?
7. Which technique do you think will be most useful—DNA probing, RFLP, or PCR—in the area of pathogenic microbiology?
8. Compare the specificity of DNA probing, RFLP, and PCR.

Student Questions

Case 9 Antibiotics

Hillary, a 2-year-old girl, had otitis media due to a *Streptococcus pneumoniae* infection acquired 6 months ago. That infection had been successfully treated with penicillin. Now her mother noted that Hillary was once again showing all the symptoms of a middle ear infection. Fortunately there was still a little penicillin left from Hillary's earlier illness, so her mother treated her for 2 days with the remainder of the medication. After the penicillin supply was exhausted, Hillary's mother noted that her daughter hadn't shown much improvement, so she took Hillary to the pediatrician.

The pediatrician took material from the ear for bacteriologic cultures and began Hillary on ampicillin. The next day the cultures were reported as "No pathogens found."

Questions

1. What are penicillin binding proteins?
2. Describe beta lactamases.
3. How did Hillary's treatment favor the proliferation of antibiotic-resistant bacteria?
4. What is the site of action of penicillin?
5. What is the site of action of ampicillin?
6. What other antibiotics act at this site?
7. If the ear cultures were negative, should ampicillin treatment be stopped?
8. How do cephalosporins differ from penicillins?
9. What are second-, third-, and fourth-generation beta-lactam agents?
10. Is penicillin resistance always plasmid mediated?

Student Questions

Case 10 Urine Count

Brenda, a 26-year-old woman, came to the emergency department at 9 PM with a complaint of lower back pain and a burning sensation during urination. She had these complaints for about 4 days and would have come for medical treatment sooner, but she had been taking some penicillin left over from an illness of one of her children. Her vital signs were all within the normal range, and the diagnosis was apparent.

A clean-catch urine sample was collected and sent to the laboratory with a provisional diagnosis of pyelonephritis.

Questions

1. What bacteria are frequently identified in pyelonephritis?
2. What is the basis of the dipstick tests for bacteriuria?
3. Describe the value of 10^5 bacteria/ml of urine recovered in culture as proof of a urinary tract infection.
4. What is the value of Gram stains of the sediment of centrifuged urine?
5. Are agents of pyelonephritis of endogenous or exogenous origin?
6. Which agents of pyelonephritis are gram-positive and potentially sensitive to penicillin?
7. Does an alkaline pH of urine greater than 8 suggest any particular pathogen?
8. What culture media are recommended for urine cultures?
9. What therapy would you choose if a gram-negative organism is isolated?
10. What does the failure of a penicillin self-cure suggest to you about the etiology of this case?

Student Questions

Review Questions

1. Which of the following antibiotics acts at the 50S ribosome level of bacteria?
   A. Streptomycin
   B. Chloramphenicol
   C. Carbapenems
   D. Tetracycline
   E. Polymyxin

2. Penicillin binding proteins are
   A. Not produced in penicillin tolerant cells
   B. All beta lactamases
   C. Enzymes found in the cytoplasmic membrane of gram positive bacteria
   D. Unable to bind second- or third-generation penicillin derivatives
   E. Also known as cell wall autolysins

3. A chemotherapeutic useful in the treatment of trichomoniasis and infections caused by gram-negative anaerobes is
   A. Griseofulvin
   B. Isoniazid (INH)
   C. Metronidazole
   D. Nalidixic acid
   E. Sulfamethoxazole

4. Which of the following chemotherapeutics influences bacterial DNA structure?
   A. Chloramphenicol
   B. Vancomycin
   C. Erythromycin
   D. Streptomycin
   E. Quinolones

5. A pure culture of chloramphenicol-sensitive *Escherichia coli* is inoculated into a broth medium containing chloramphenicol. After 18 hours of growth on a shaking apparatus, samples of the broth were streaked onto an agar medium containing chloramphenicol, and several colonies then grew. The resistant cells probably arose

   A. Because chloramphenicol induces mutations
   B. By conjugation of F^+ resistant with F^- sensitive cells
   C. By transformation
   D. By mutation and selection
   E. By transduction

6. Which of the structures of the bacterial cell is affected by tetracyclines?

   A. Peptidoglycan
   B. DNA
   C. Folic acid synthesis
   D. 30S ribosome
   E. Cytoplasmic membrane

7. Which of the following is considered more effective against gram-negative bacteria than against gram-positive bacteria?

   A. Polymyxin
   B. Penicillin
   C. Erythromycin
   D. Cephalosporins
   E. Isoniazid

8. Which of the following contains a dihydrothiazine ring?

   A. Penicillin
   B. Chloramphenicol
   C. Clavulanic acid
   D. Monobactams
   E. Cephalosporin

9. Cyloserine

   A. Blocks the carrier activity of bactoprenol by combining with its phosphate grouping
   B. Is effective against mycoplasma
   C. Inhibits alanine racemase
   D. Is a structural analog of phosphoenolpyruvate
   E. Is inactivated by the addition of adenyl groups

10. The best combination from the following list for treating tuberculosis is

    A. Penicillin and sulfamethoxazole
    B. Erythromycin and chloramphenicol
    C. Streptomycin and erythromycin
    D. Sulfamethoxazole and trimethoprim
    E. Isoniazid and streptomycin

3 Respiratory Tract Infections

Infections of the respiratory tract are generally considered separately as either upper or lower respiratory infections. The former are usually less serious and include rhinitis, pharyngitis, tonsillitis, epiglottitis, and laryngeotracheitis (croup). The latter, however, may be quite serious. Lower respiratory infections include bronchitis and pneumonia, both of which may be severe.

Upper respiratory infections (URI's), such as the common cold and sinusitis, are most frequently caused by viruses, a factor that often precludes an exact identification of the etiologic agent (Table 3-1). Upper respiratory infections are also caused by group A *Streptococcus pyogenes*, the common bacterial agent that causes septic sore throat.

Lower respiratory tract agents include numerous bacteria, several fungi, mycoplasma, the tubercle bacillus, and viruses, of which the influenza virus is well known for its ability to cause epidemic disease (Table 3-2). Some authors prefer to classify the pneumonias as either community or hospital acquired, recognizing that there is

Table 3-1. Viruses causing respiratory infections

		Respiratory Infection		
Agent	Classification	Upper	Lower	Comments
Adenovirus	More than 80 serologic types	Rhinitis, pharyngitis	Bronchitis, pneumonia	Also causes intestinal disease
Coxsackie virus	Types A and B	Pharyngitis	Pleurodynia	
Herpes simplex virus	HSV1 and HSV2	Pharyngitis	Bronchitis, pneumonia	Many other diseases possible
Influenza viruses	Types A, B, and C	Rhinitis, pharyngitis	Pneumonia	Vaccine available A most common
Parainfluenza	Types 1, 2, 3, and 4	Rhinitis, pharyngitis, croup	Pneumonia	Less common than influenza viruses
Respiratory syncytial virus	Types A and B	Rhinitis, croup	Pneumonia	Often targets young children
Rhinoviruses	More than 115 serotypes	Rhinitis	Very rare	About 38% of all respiratory infections

Table 3-2. Important agents other than viruses that cause respiratory infections

Agent	Classification	Infection	Key features
Bacteroides species	Gram-negative anaerobe	Aspiration pneumonia	Aged patients, alcoholics
Chlamydia pneumoniae	Bacterium	Atypical pneumonia	
Chlamydia psittaci	Bacterium	Atypical pneumonia	A zoonosis
Coccidioides immitis	Fungus	Pneumonia	Endemic in southwestern United States
Coxiella burnetii	Rickettsia	Pneumonia	Endemic in southwestern United States
Haemophilus influenzae	Bacterium, seven capsular types	Community pneumonia	Type b causes most disease, vaccine available
Histoplasma capsulatum	Fungus	Pneumonia	Endemic in central United States
Legionella pneumophila	Bacterium, many types	Pneumonia	Other species involved, immunocompromised patients
Mycobacterium tuberculosis	Acid-fast bacterium	Tuberculosis	OT and PPD skin tests, BCG vaccine
Mycoplasma pneumoniae	Cell wall–less bacterium	Atypical pneumonia	Affects primarily children
Pneumocystis carinii	Protozoan?	Pneumonia	Key disease of AIDS patients
Streptococcus pneumoniae	Bacterium, > 80 capsular types	Commonest cause of community pneumonia	Rusty sputum, effective vaccine
Streptococcus pyogenes	Bacterium, many serologic types	Pharyngitis, tonsillitis, etc.	Group A most common

not a clear distinction between these. Even so, *Streptococcus pneumoniae, Haemophilus influenzae,* and *Staphylococcus aureus* are more likely to appear in the first rather than the second group. The second group includes pneumonias due to *Klebsiella, Pseudomonas*, and *Legionella,* but many other gram-negative bacteria could be listed here, particularly in aged or immunocompromised patients. Aspiration pneumonia is a special category of pneumonia seen often but not exclusively in hospitalized patients. *Bacteroides* species, staphylococci, and gram-negative bacilli are often encountered in this type of pneumonia. Chronic pneumonia may be caused by the tubercle bacillus and related mycobacteria, several fungi, a few parasites, and *Pneumocystis carinii.*

Radiographic features of pneumonias rarely identify a single etiology. Examination of sputum by direct staining and culture, and blood cultures are the most frequently used and successful diagnostic tests. Transtracheal aspiration may be needed to recover pathogens from patients who are critically ill, especially where anaerobes are suspected. Serologic tests, requiring both acute and convalescent sera, are needed to diagnose pneumonias caused by viruses or mycoplasma.

Key Words and Phrases

After a careful study of the cases in this chapter and related conditions, you should be able to describe the meaning and use of the following abbreviations, words, and phrases.

Acid-fast
Antigenic drift
Antigenic shift
Arthroconidia
Arthrospores
Aspiration pneumonia
Atypical acid-fast organism
Atypical pneumonia
Carrier
Cold agglutinin
Cord factor
Dimorphic fungus
Droplet nuclei
Endospores
Fried egg colony
Hemagglutination inhibition
Hemagglutinin
Microconidia
Mold phase
Mycolic acid
Neuraminidase
Niacin production test
Nitrate reductase test
Optochin
Photochromogen
Polyvalent pneumococcal vaccine
Q fever
Reye's syndrome
Sabouraud's medium
Scotochromogen
Spherule
Split virus vaccine
Tuberculate macroconidia (chlamydospores)
Walking pneumonia
Yeast phase

Abbreviations

BCG	OT
HSV	PPD
MAC	RSV

Information Sources

Bluestone, C.D., and Klein, S.O.: Otitis media in infants and children, W.B. Saunders Co., 1988, Philadelphia.

Easmon, C.S.F., editor: Staphylococci and staphylococcal disease, Academic Press, Inc., 1983, New York.

Finegold, S.M.: Anaerobic bacteria in human disease, Academic Press, Inc., 1977, New York.

Grange, J.M.: Mycobacteria and human disease, Edward Arnold, 1988, London.

Heffron, R.: Pneumonia, Harvard University Press, 1979, Cambridge.

Kilbourne, E.D.: Influenza, Plenum Medical Book Co., 1987, New York.

Mandell, G.L., Douglas, R.G., Jr., and Bennett, E., editors: Principles and practice of infectious diseases, edition 3, Churchill Livingstone, 1990, New York.

Maniloff, J., editor: Mycoplasmas, ASM Press, 1992, Herndon, VA.

Marrie, T.J., editor: Q fever: the disease, vol. 1, CRC Press, 1990, Boca Raton.

Pennington, J.E., editor: Respiratory infections: diagnosis and management, edition 2, Raven Press, 1989, New York.

Read, S.E., and Zabriskie, J.M., editors: Streptococcal diseases and the immune response, Academic Press, Inc., 1980, Orlando.

Remington, J.S., and Klein, J.O.: Infectious diseases of the fetus and newborn infant, edition 3, W.B. Saunders Co., 1990, Philadelphia.

Roizman, B., Whitely, R.J., and Lopez, C., editors: The human herpes viruses, Raven Press, 1993, New York.

Sarosi, G.A., and Davies, S.F., editors: Fungal diseases of the lung, Raven Press, 1993, New York.

Schlossberg, D., editor: Infectious mononucleosis, edition 2, Springer-Verlag, 1989, New York.

Schoolnik, G.K.: The pathogenic neisseriae, American Society for Microbiology, 1985, Washington.

Wardlaw, A.C., and Parton, R.: Pathogenesis and immunity in pertussis, John Wiley and Sons, 1988, New York.

Case 1 A Mistaken Diagnosis of Cancer

Jack R., a UCLA graduate, had been a professor of biochemistry in an Arkansas medical school for 4 years. Each summer he and his family made the long drive from Little Rock to Los Angeles to visit their families. This year the return trip had been a little more adventurous. Jack and his wife decided to spend a few evenings camping out in some of the national parks along the way.

On the evening of August 5, they arrived at a park in western Arizona only to find that it was already filled. The park guide directed them to a privately owned campground only 5 miles away. The owner and his wife were very pleased to meet them and offered a generous breakfast as part of their camping fee. During the night a severe dust storm nearly took down the family tent, but the next morning the family showered in the camp facility, repacked their car, and enjoyed their breakfast of biscuits, eggs, sausage, coffee, and their first taste of goat's milk from the campground owner's herd.

Three months later, back in Arkansas, Jack's annual medical examination included a chest x-ray, after which Jack was operated on for cancer. Histopathologic examination of lung tissue revealed that the diagnosis of cancer had been made in error.

Questions

1. What infectious disease(s) of the lung could be confused with lung cancer?
2. Can this disease be acquired from goat's milk?
3. Is this disease endemic in Arkansas, Los Angeles, or anywhere between?
4. What do you think is the source of Jack's disease? Are animals a reservoir for this agent?
5. What special resistance does this agent have that enables it to survive in a hostile environment?
6. What is the appearance of this pathogen in culture?
7. How would you culture this agent?
8. What special precautions should be taken with these cultures?
9. What is the appearance of this pathogen in vivo?
10. Why is it that Jack never complained of any illness the entire time he had this disease?
11. Is this an agent that appears to be more virulent for certain racial groups than others?
12. What forms do acute infections with this agent take?
13. Are skin tests useful in diagnosing this disease? Explain.
14. What serologic test(s) could be used to diagnose this disease?
15. How is acute infection with this agent treated?

Student Questions

Case 2 The Nursing Home

Harvey W. was a 78-year-old resident of a nursing care home for the elderly. He had lived in the home for the past 3 years because of incapacitation due to Alzheimer's disease. He had adjusted quite well to life in the nursing home and with assistance was able to dress himself, bathe, and take care of his daily hygienic needs. Meals were taken with other retirees in a common dining room. Harvey enjoyed the recreation room, not because he could play cards, paint, or enjoy other hobbies, but because it was the only place in the building where he and other smokers could enjoy their habit (under close supervision).

In early July, construction for a new wing on the nursing home was begun. The addition would consist of a ward built parallel to the area where Harvey lived but with adequate space between the two wings for the patients to have a small flower garden and shade tree area. The new area would have central, rather than individual window air-conditioning as in the older part of the building where Harvey lived. Harvey was excited by the construction activity only a few feet outside his window, where he stood for hours each day watching the workers using their earth-moving equipment.

As the nurse made her early morning rounds on July 15, she noticed that Harvey, who refused to get up from bed, had a cough. She determined that his temperature was 102.6°F. The home's private physician was called and after auscultation determined that Harvey had pneumonia in the lower lobes of both lungs. Harvey was transported to the hospital, where x-rays confirmed the pneumonia. It was impossible to collect sputum for bacteriologic studies because of increasing confusion of the patient.

Erythromycin was prescribed, but before the central pharmacy could transfer the antibiotic to his hospital room, Harvey suddenly became comatose and cyanotic, and he expired. Harvey's family had been summoned and gave authorization for an autopsy. Lung tissue yielded *Enterobacter aerogenes* on blood agar plates but in low numbers after 24 hours of culture. No other potential pathogens were recovered. Blood cultures were heavily contaminated and rendered useless by *Bacillus* species. A serum sample was sent to the State Health Laboratory for serologic studies.

Questions

1. What etiologic agents are associated with a fulminating pneumonia like that seen here?
2. Are these agents particularly prone to infect the aged?
3. Are these agents particularly prevalent in nursing homes, hospitals, and other health care centers?
4. Does your answer to question 3 implicate health care workers or other residents of the home as carriers of the agents, or are these opportunistic, indigenous, or environmental agents?
5. Is *Enterobacter aerogenes* your sole consideration as the pathogen in this case? Explain this in relation to the low numbers recovered.

6. What potential bacteriologic agents of pneumonia would not be recovered after 24 hours of culture?
7. Which of your answers to question 6 suggest an environmental source? A carrier source?
8. Regarding a potential environmental source, are any of these soil-borne organisms?
9. What culture conditions are required to recover highly fastidious pathogens that cause fulminating pneumonia in the aged?
10. What serologic tests are useful in identifying these agents?
11. What cultural characteristics are useful in recovering these agents from tissue?
12. What is the immune status in patients who survive this disease?

Student Questions

Case 3 A Mild Pneumonia

Carrie and Claudia were sisters, ages 15 and 17, who attended the same high school. Their 12-year-old brother Carl went to junior high school. The girls shared the same bedroom but slept in separate beds. Carl had his own bedroom. The childrens' and parents' bedrooms were on separate floors of the house. The children shared one bathroom and the parents a second. The family normally ate their morning and evening meals together on weekdays, the children having their lunch at school. On weekends, eating times were haphazard except for Sunday dinner, which the family usually ate together.

On Friday, June 12, the last day of school, Carl came home complaining of a sore throat. On Saturday, his throat was really bothering him. He also had a postnasal drip and cough. His mother took his temperature, which was 100.4°F. She gave Carl aspirin to reduce his fever and antihistamines to slow his postnasal drip. When she insisted that Carl miss the soccer game, he was too tired to argue, and he remained indoors most of the day. Carl's condition remained essentially the same for the next week—a slight fever, cough, excessive malaise, and headache. During the following week, Carl began to feel much better, although he did not lose his cough.

Unfortunately, it was just at this time that his mother developed what seemed to be the same illness—sore throat, headache, cough, and excessive malaise. Two days later when both Carrie and Claudia came down with it, their mother, determined to find the cause of this illness, took both daughters to their doctor.

The doctor's diagnosis was a mild pneumonia of uncertain cause. He collected throat swabs from both girls for bacteriologic studies in his clinic's small laboratory. Blood samples were also collected from the two girls for antibody studies. He started the girls on erythromycin.

The next day the physician's secretary called to say that the girls had normal throat cultures and that the results of the antibody studies wouldn't be available until next week, since it was necessary to send the blood to a central laboratory. The mother told the secretary that her husband seemed to be coming down with the same disease and she would like to know what was going on as soon as the doctor found out.

Questions

1. What etiologic agents are associated with a highly contagious, relatively mild pneumonia?
2. Since Carrie and Claudia had normal throat cultures, does this limit your consideration to viral agents?
3. What bacteria could be missed by routine culturing of throat swabs?
4. Notice that this physician did not do a rapid serologic test for streptococci. Why?
5. Does this family group meet the general description of having walking pneumonia?
6. What are the agents of walking pneumonia? Describe their unique characteristics.
7. Which of the pathogens listed in your answer to question 6 is sensitive to erythromycin?
8. Why didn't the physician prescribe penicillin for this community-acquired pneumonia?
9. What serologic tests could be useful in diagnosing this disease? Describe such tests.
10. Explain how DNA probes could be used to diagnose this disease.
11. What organisms are considered part of the normal throat flora?

Student Questions

Case 4 An Overworked Student

Some people said that Ellen was more like a man than a woman. She lived alone in a ramshackle house in the country, a house that lacked central heating and running water. Ellen cut her own firewood right on the acreage. She pumped water from a well that was installed under the kitchen. Three or four vagrant dogs were her only company. This isolation was in far contrast to her upbringing in the tenements in Chicago. There the noise, the pollution, and near starvation led many black kids like her to drugs, death, or jail.

Ellen had battled against all this with a determination unusual in her neighborhood. She received a minority fellowship to go to college, and after that her grade point and Graduate Record Examination scores got her a research assistantship in the Department of Biochemistry. The pay wasn't much, but at least she would be able to get her Ph.D.

For the last 5 months Ellen had been doing triple duty. She still had her biochemistry laboratory section to teach, and she was trying to polish up some of her research experiments. In addition, her advisor wanted the Introduction and Materials and Methods sections of her dissertation finished before spring break.

Over the last 2 months, Ellen could feel herself wearing down. She felt so tired at 9 or 10 at night that she had to close the laboratory and head home. The extra hour or two of sleep each night didn't seem to help. She had lost almost 10 pounds, which at first she attributed to poor eating habits. Now that she was having mild night sweats and an occasional fever, she felt it was time to visit the student health clinic.

Her laboratory findings were unremarkable—normal leukocyte count, normal blood and urine chemistry. Physical data were more revealing, especially the chest plates that revealed a nodular infiltration and possible cavitation of her left lung. She was skin tested with PPD and was asked to bring up some sputum for culturing.

Questions

1. Which of these environmental factors are predisposing to Ellen's illness—well water, canine pets, early poverty in the tenements, stress from overwork, or poor diet?
2. What respiratory illnesses are linked to the environmental factors listed in question 1? Are any of these diseases latent?
3. Nodular deposits in the lung suggest at least two obvious respiratory diseases. Name two agents and describe their major characteristics.
4. Do cavitary lesions in the lung eliminate either of these diseases?
5. Why was PPD rather than OT used in the skin test?
6. How are reactions to PPD evaluated?
7. What other skin tests could be suggested here?
8. What are your recommendations for culturing the sputum?
9. Describe specific staining and biochemical tests that would be useful here.
10. How would the use of Southern blotting accelerate the diagnosis?
11. What therapy would you recommend for your diagnosis (or diagnoses)?
12. Why are (or aren't) you advising combination therapy?

Student Questions

Case 5 Pneumonia

Doc Rigney remembered Harold as a young man and then later as the owner of his own construction company. Harold was a person who simply wouldn't heed good advice. Take the automobile accident as an example. Only 2 months after receiving his driver's license, he crashed his Dad's car. A broken nose, facial lacerations, a few minor cuts and bruises, plus a ruptured spleen that had to be removed slowed him down for several weeks. Most of this could have been prevented if he had been wearing his seat belt.

Then there was the ice-skating incident his first year at college. Despite signs posted at the golf course lake that the ice was unsafe, he convinced his girlfriend that they should go for a moonlight skate. They were fortunate to get out alive but only because they broke through at the shallow end of the lake.

Doc also remembered Harold's retirement vacation trip to Indonesia last year when Harold refused to take a gamma globulin shot against hepatitis. Sure enough he got it, probably from eating food offered by street vendors.

And now Harold was in the hospital with pneumonia. Doc Rigney's son, Doc Junior, was taking care of him. It was a typical case—fever 102°F, cough of 3 days' duration, chills, slight lower right chest pain, and a rusty sputum. Why hadn't Harold taken the vaccine that both Doc Senior and Doc Junior had recommended?

Questions

1. What symptom(s) should lead you to the correct diagnosis of this form of pneumonia?
2. Discuss the organism involved here.
3. Is this agent ever a part of the normal flora?
4. What vaccine had the doctors advised? Discuss its composition and use.
5. Does Harold have any special predisposition to this form of pneumonia?
6. What other major illnesses are caused by the agent causing this pneumonia?
7. Discuss hemolysis caused by bacteria on blood agar plates.

8. What laboratory techniques are used to identify this pathogen?
9. What is the C-reactive protein, and how does it relate to this case?
10. What kind of hepatitis did Harold contract in Indonesia?
11. Describe the etiologic agents of viral hepatitis.

Student Questions

Case 6 One Too Many

Eric, a 32-year-old alcoholic, was well-known to the emergency room staff. In the past 6 or 8 months they had seen Eric for a drug overdose, pneumococcal pneumonia, and a broken nose suffered in an alley fight. Eric was a homeless alcoholic who slept in door fronts or wherever he could until he finally assembled some cartons and sheet metal to fashion his own "home."

Once again Eric was brought in by the police ambulance. Eric's friends had become alarmed when he didn't come out of his cardboard shack all day, and by evening they went to investigate. Eric was semidelerious and had an obvious fever and a bad cough. His raglike handkerchief was wet with sputum. It was then that they contacted the police.

On admission, Eric presented as an underweight man in obvious respiratory distress. Chest sounds of the posterior upper right lobe were consistent with pneumonia, and an x-ray confirmed this. While Eric was in a state of consciousness it was possible to take his temperature (102.2°F), collect sputum for bacteriologic culture, and take a sample of blood (87% neutrophils and a count of 11,400). Eric was hospitalized and given clindamycin. The next day the laboratory reported normal respiratory flora.

Questions

1. What, if any, respiratory infections are associated with a drug overdose?
2. What, if any, respiratory infections are associated with alcoholism?
3. Do the chest sounds or x-ray suggest any particular pathogen(s)?
4. What are the criteria of a good sputum sample for bacteriologic analysis?

5. Are normal respiratory flora ever involved in pneumonia?
6. Is there significance in the choice of clindamycin as the antibiotic?
7. What dangers are associated with the use of clindamycin?
8. Describe the differences between community-acquired, hospital-acquired, and aspiration pneumonia.
9. How does the etiology of these three pneumonias differ?
10. What are the agents of chronic pneumonia?
11. How can anaerobic bacteria live in the lung and cause pneumonia?
12. Describe methods of creating anaerobic cultures in the laboratory.

Student Questions

Case 7 When Muriel Flew Home

Muriel realized she had returned home too soon from her winter in Florida. The snow flurries outside were evidence enough of that, but she could also feel a cold coming on.

Or maybe she was still just tired from the trip. At 79 years of age, she was pleased by the way she had navigated the airports in Atlanta and Chicago. She had to ask directions of several strangers, but most of them had been quite obliging to an old lady. The most distressful part of the trip was sitting next to that woman who couldn't stop sneezing. That was obviously the cause of all this.

Two days later Muriel realized this was not simply a cold. In the intervening 48 hours, her symptoms had progressed from some mild sneezing to a gentle and then definite headache, muscle pains, fever, and shortness of breath. She decided to call her son-in-law and have him take her to the doctor.

Dr. Finnerty noted that Muriel now had a temperature of 103.2°F and every evidence of a pneumonia. X-rays revealed an acute generalized edema. He asked Muriel if she had been given vaccines for pneumonia in Florida, and she responded affirmatively.

Questions

1. Does a minor cold "change" into influenza or pneumonia? If so, how?
2. Does a generalized edema of the lungs suggest any particular etiologic agent(s) as the cause of Muriel's pneumonia?
3. What vaccines could Muriel have taken in Florida to prevent pneumonia? Explain in detail.
4. What climatic, behavioral, or other noninfectious conditions predispose a person to pneumonia?
5. What microbiologic steps would Dr. Finnerty request to confirm the diagnosis?
6. What immunologic procedures would Dr. Finnerty request to aid in the diagnosis?
7. Just how negligent was Dr. Finnerty in not taking specimens for bacterial cultures? Does this mean he was convinced this was a case of viral pneumonia?
8. Describe three important viruses that cause lower respiratory infections.
9. Which of these are known to vary their antigenic makeup regularly?
10. How does viral pneumonia compare to pneumonia caused by rickettsia?

Student Questions

Case 8 Cleaned Up and Cleaned Out

Principal Fowler of West Madison Middle School, in a city near the Missouri River, looked at the school absence reports again. The usual 20 to 40 absences in grades 7, 8, and 9 had soared to 106 last Thursday and to 180 last Friday. This week the numbers had remained unusually high. He called the head school nurse to see if she could explain the cause of this.

Nurse Wilkinson reported that she had encountered an abnormal number of students early last week with headache, fever, and chest pain, at least half of whom had a cough and nausea. For the most part, these were the same students who were absent this week. She suggested they call the City Health Officer if this absenteeism continued throughout the week.

On the following Monday, the Health Officer visited the school and talked with Nurse Wilkinson and Principal Fowler. In an attempt to relate this incident to some activity that affected all three classes of the school equally, he noted that an all-school cleanup day had been held just 3 weeks previously. All the children had raked leaves, planted trees and flowers, sown grass seed, or were otherwise engaged in cleaning the school grounds. Children who had done the most vigorous cleaning, especially those involved in cleaning the wooded area on the other side of the athletic field, had the highest incidence of absenteeism. By the time this information was gathered and skin tests prepared for some of the students, class attendance was back to normal.

Questions

1. Is this history suggestive of legionellosis? What is Pontiac fever?
2. Is this history suggestive of other respiratory diseases?
3. What skin tests were envisioned here?
4. Wouldn't all the students be positive for these skin tests?
5. The return of class attendance back to normal in only a week eliminates what etiologic agents? Incriminates what agents?
6. Describe the growth and morphology of the agents you listed for question 5.
7. If you included a fungus in your answers to question 5, explain how the infective and the culture forms of these fungi differ.
8. Which pneumonias are contagious, and which are not?
9. You probably didn't include respiratory diseases caused by animal parasites in your answer to question 8. How do certain worms cause respiratory complaints?
10. Will the affected children in this case have good immunity against reinfection?

Student Questions

Case 9 A Double Dose

Harold G., a known alcoholic, was a 53-year-old factory employee who had just returned to work after a 3-week sick leave due to an influenza A infection. On his first day back, he still felt somewhat weak, and by mid-afternoon he began to develop a dry, rough cough. He continued to work the next 2 days, but by the end of the second day he had intermittent fever and chills and chest pain. He told his foreman that he was going to visit the company physician. While in the waiting room, he had a prolonged coughing spell and brought up a thick, rust-colored sputum.

The physician's findings were as follows:

Temperature	102.2°F
Pulse	86
Respiration	39, shallow
Blood pressure	158/87 mm Hg

The patient was pale and sweaty, appeared in acute distress, and continued to cough.

Laboratory findings showed 8500 white blood cells/mm^3. Chest x-ray revealed a diffuse patchy infiltrate in the right middle and lower lobes. A Gram stain of the sputum contained gram-positive cocci in clusters.

Questions

1. What are the most common bacterial causes of pneumonia in adults?
2. What, if any, is the relationship of alcoholism and an antecedent influenza infection to a bacterial pneumonia?
3. Are gram-positive cocci in clusters invariably staphylococci?
4. What is the expected course of staphylococcal pneumonia?
5. What is the recommended therapy of staphylococcal infections?
6. What is the basis of antibiotic resistance in staphylococci?
7. What features are used to distinguish pathogenic staphylococci from non-pathogenic strains and from closely related genera?
8. Is a rust-colored sputum an important key in this diagnosis?
9. Should acid-fast stains of sputum be considered in this case?
10. What is the epidemiologic significance of an influenza type A infection in this case?
11. How are influenza viruses identified?
12. Describe reassortment of influenza viruses.
13. Explain antigenic drift and antigenic shift of the influenza viruses.

Student Questions

Review Questions

1. Which of the following diseases is caused by an etiologic agent with a complex intracellular life cycle?
   A. Leptospirosis
   B. Legionnaire's disease
   C. Psittacosis
   D. Pertussis
   E. Syphilis

2. Which of the following cell wall constituents of *Staphylococcus aureus* binds to the Fc fragment of immunoglobulin G?
   A. Capsular polysaccharide
   B. Lipopolysaccharide
   C. Peptidoglycan
   D. Protein A
   E. Teichoic acid

3. Which of the following characteristics is **not** associated with mycoplasmas?
   A. "Fried egg" colony morphology
   B. Cold agglutinin test
   C. Penicillin sensitivity
   D. Pleomorphism
   E. Sterol requirement

4. Pathogenicity of group A, beta-hemolytic streptococci seems **best** correlated with the production of
   A. C carbohydrate
   B. Hyaluronic acid capsule
   C. M protein
   D. Streptokinase
   E. Streptolysin S

5. The **least** useful procedure for diagnosis of Legionnaire's disease is
   A. Culture
   B. Animal inoculation
   C. Gram stain
   D. Immunofluorescence
   E. Microagglutination

6. The constituent of *Streptococcus pneumoniae* that determines both its virulence and specific type is the
   A. Capsular polysaccharide
   B. Cell wall carbohydrate
   C. Flagellar protein

D. Nucleoprotein structure
E. Thermal leukocidin

7. All six men who cleared a field of bamboo cane in Louisiana developed pulmonary disease within 6 to 14 days. The field was known to be a blackbird roosting site, and the ground in the middle of the field was covered with droppings. During the first 5 to 7 days of the illness, the primary symptoms were abdominal cramps and diarrhea followed by rising fever, cough, chest pain, and dyspnea. Chest x-rays showed widespread miliary infiltration. One patient developed respiratory failure and was treated with amphotericin B and recovered. The others recovered without specific therapy. These findings are consistent with an etiology of

A. *Actinomyces israelii*
B. *Candida albicans*
C. *Histoplasma capsulatum*
D. *Mycobacterium tuberculosis*
E. *Sporothrix schenckii*

8. The etiologic agent of histoplasmosis is a

A. Multiple budding yeast
B. Sclerotic cell
C. Yeast
D. Spherule/endospore-producing fungus
E. None of the above is correct

9. The capsule of group A streptococci

A. Can be detected by the Francis test
B. Is a good candidate for a protective vaccine
C. Is degraded by hyaluronidase
D. Is an adhesin
E. None of the above is correct

10. Vaccination against pneumococci is recommended for

A. Premature infants
B. Expectant mothers
C. Patients with lobar pneumonia
D. Rheumatic fever patients
E. Asplenic patients

11. The utility of skin tests in the diagnosis of histoplasmosis is hampered by

A. The cross-reactivity of histoplasmin in other systemic fungal diseases
B. The high incidence of infection without disease in large areas of the central United States
C. The fact that a person once positive in response to histoplasmin will normally remain positive for many years
D. The fact that histoplasmin is antigenic and its use can interfere with a serologic diagnosis of histoplasmosis
E. All of the above are correct

12. With one exception, all of the following function as adhesins of *Staphylococcus aureus*. The exception is

A. Lipoteichoic acid
B. Bound coagulase
C. Clumping factor
D. Exfoliatin
E. Protein A

13. *Mycobacterium tuberculosis* is very resistant to chemical agents, drying, and basic dyes due to

A. Endospore formation
B. The high lipid content of its cell wall
C. Lack of a cell wall
D. A polysaccharide capsule
E. Its inability to grow outside host cells

14. A positive test for cold agglutinins in a patient with pneumonia is presumptive evidence of infection with

A. *Streptococcus pneumoniae*
B. *Mycoplasma pneumoniae*
C. *Klebsiella pneumoniae*
D. Influenza virus
E. Adenovirus

15. Which of the following tests is used to measure immunity to influenza virus?

A. Antigenic drift
B. Hemagglutination
C. Complement fixation with split vaccine as the antigen
D. Passive hemagglutination inhibition
E. Hemagglutination inhibition

4 Food- and Water-Borne Diseases

Acute infectious diarrhea is the leading cause of disease and death in many areas of the world. Each primary care physician in North America is estimated to encounter 200 cases of acute gastroenteritis annually. Among illnesses affecting families, acute gastroenteritis is second only to the common cold.

Diarrhea is usually defined as the excretion of greater than 300g of stool daily with increased liquidity and frequency. There are many causes of diarrhea. The most common causes of acute infectious diarrheas are presumed to be of viral origin. Even with sophisticated techniques, the specific etiology of acute diarrhea illness is established only about 50% of the time and, in clinical practice, is determined only 10% to 20% of the time. The etiologic agents may be bacteria, bacterial toxins, or animal parasites in addition to viruses. Fungi are less frequently involved.

The following tables summarize information about bacterial intoxications and bacterial infections as sources of acute diarrhea. In bacterial intoxications, the toxin is present in the food when it is consumed (Table 4-1). In bacterial infections, the organisms entering in food or water must proliferate before they can cause disease (Table 4-2). They may do this by producing toxins or by other means as the bacteria grow, but this takes time. Because of this difference, food-borne intoxications have a shorter incubation time than most infections.

Most cases of infectious diarrhea are caused by viruses (Table 4-3). It is estimated that the rotaviruses cause 3.5 million cases of diarrhea per year in the United States and 140 million cases worldwide. Rarely are viruses ever recovered and identified except in large outbreaks or academic studies of diarrhea. Often the etiology can be intimated by the nature (age) of the patient group or by the nature of the illness (incubation time, symptoms, epidemiology). Since therapy of viral diarrheas is symptomatic, knowledge of the exact etiology is often of little value.

Intestinal parasites may cause a transient or chronic diarrhea (Table 4-4).

Table 4-1. Gastroenteritis due to food-borne intoxications

					Clinical Features			
Organism	Reservoir	Vehicle	Toxin	Incubation	Vomiting	Abdominal Cramps	Diarrhea	Duration
Bacillus cereus	Soil	Fried rice	Preformed	1–6 hours	++++	++	+	6–12 hours
		(others)	Luminal production	8–16 hours	+	++++	++++	24 hours
Campylobacter jejuni	Soil, animals	Water, food	Luminal production	1–7 days	+	+	++	24 hours or chronic
Clostridium difficile	Man, animals	None	Luminal production	Variable	+	+++	+++	Variable
Clostridium perfringens	Soil	Cooked meat (others)	Luminal production	8–16 hours	+	++++	++++	24 hours
*Escherichia coli**	Man, animals	Water	Luminal production	4–24 hours	+	+	++++	1–3 days
Staphylococcus aureus	Man	Many foods	Preformed (heat stable)	1–6 hours	++++	++	+	6–12 hours
Vibrio cholerae	Man, shellfish	Water	Luminal production	6–72 hours	+	0	++++	2–5 days

*Enterotoxic *E. coli* (ETEC); see Table 4-2 for enteropathogenic *E. coli.*

Table 4-2. Gastroenteritis due to food-borne infections

Organism	Reservoir	Vehicle	Mucosal Penetration	Incubation	Clinical Features	Duration
Escherichia coli[a]	Man	Water	No[b]	1–3 days	Dysentery	1–3 days
Helicobacter pylori	Man	Water, milk	Yes	2–4 days	Dysentery	3–5 days
Salmonella enteriditis[c]	Animal	Food (poultry)	Occasionally	8–48 hours	Diarrhea	1–3 days
Salmonella typhi	Man	Water or food	Yes	1–3 weeks	Fever, constipation, diarrhea, skin rash, pharyngitis, etc.	Relapses 10–20%
Shigella sonnei and other species	Man	Human, fecal-oral	No[b]	1–3 days	Bloody diarrhea	3–6 days
Vibrio parahaemolyticus[d]	Salt water	Shellfish	Yes	4–48 hours	Watery diarrhea	12–72 hours
Yersinia enterocolitica	Animals	Water	Yes	1–10 days	Dysentery, acute appendicitis, mesenteric adenitis	2 days

[a]Enteropathogenic *E. coli* (EPEC) and others.
[b]Invades and destroys epithelium (rarely causes bacteremia).
[c]Many other species and serotypes.
[d]Also produces enterotoxins but role in pathogenesis unclear.

Table 4-3. Common viral agents of diarrhea

Virus	Target Group	Incubation Time	Symptoms
Adenovirus types 40 and 41	< 2 years old	3–10 days	Diarrhea about 1 week
Astrovirus	< 7 years old	1–1½ days	Diarrhea 1–4 days
Calicivirus	Children	1–3 days	Diarrhea about 4 days
Enterovirus, echovirus	All age groups	3–5 days	Other aspects of disease (e.g.,Coxsackie virus) more serious
Norwalk agent	School age–adult	2–4 days	Diarrhea 12 hours–5 days
Rotavirus	6 months–2 years	2 days	Vomiting about 3 days, diarrhea 3–8 days, very contagious

Table 4-4. Gastroenteritis due to animal parasites*

Organism	Reservoir	Vehicle	Clinical Features
Balantidium coli	Pigs	Water, food	Diarrhea, intestinal ulceration
Cryptosporidium parvum	Man, domestic animals	Water, food	Watery diarrhea
Entamoeba histolytica	Man	Water, fresh foods	Dysentery, secondary amebiasis
Giardia lamblia	Man	Water	Explosive diarrhea, malabsorption
Isospora belli	Man	Water, food	Chronic diarrhea

*Many helminths may cause abdominal infections with pain and/or diarrhea (e.g., *Trichina*, *Taenia*, *Ancylostoma*, *Necator*). In addition, other animal parasites (e.g., *Toxoplasma*, *Plasmodium*, *Schistosoma*) may cause intestinal disease.

Key Words and Phrases

The key words, phrases, and abbreviations for this chapter have been divided into four subheadings appropriate for the study of food- and water-borne diseases.

MEDIA

EMB agar
Hektoen enteric agar
IMViC test
MacConkey agar
Selenite broth
SS agar
Tetrathionate broth
TSI agar

TOXINS

A-B type toxin
Adenylate cyclase
ADP ribosyl transferase
Choleragen
Choleragenoid
C *tox*
Cyclic AMP
Cytotoxin
Enterotoxin
GM I ganglioside
LT
Shiga toxin
ST

ILLNESS

Diarrhea
Dysentery
Food poisoning
Infant botulism
Necrotizing entercolitis
Oral rehydration salts
Pseudomembranous colitis
Tenesmus
Traveler's diarrhea

AGENTS

Calicivirus
CFA
Coliform
Coronavirus
Cyst
EHEC
EIEC
EPEC
ETEC
H antigen
K antigen
Lactose fermenter
Norwalk agent
O antigen
Rotavirus
Trophozoite
Vi antigen

Information Sources

Bock, G., and Whelan, J., editors: Novel diarrhoea viruses, Wiley-Interscience, 1987, Chichester.

Butzler, J.P., editor: *Campylobacter* infections in man and animals, CRC Press, 1984, Boca Raton.

Cook, G.C.: Parasitic disease in clinical practice, Springer-Verlag, 1990, New York.

Doyle, M.P., editor: Foodborne bacterial pathogens, Marcel Dekker, Inc., 1989, New York.

DuPont, H.L., and Pickering, L.K.: Infections of the gastrointestinal tract, microbiology, pathophysiology, and clinical features, Plenum Press, 1980, New York.

Ellner, P.D., editor: Infectious diarrheal diseases: current concepts and laboratory procedures, Marcel Dekker, Inc., 1984, New York.

Evered, D., and Whelan, J., editors: Microbial toxins and diarrhoeal disease, Pittman, 1985, London.

Field, M., editor: Diarrheal diseases, Elsevier Science Publishing Co., Inc., 1991, New York.

Gorbach, S.L., editor: Infectious diarrhea, Blackwell Scientific Publications, Inc., 1986, Boston.

Gust, I.D., and Feinstone, S.M., editors: Hepatitis A, CRC Press, 1989, Boca Raton.

Hollinger, F.B., editor: Viral hepatitis: biological and clinical features, Raven Press, 1991, New York.

Holmgren, J., Lindberg, A., and Mollby, R., editors: Development of vaccines and drugs against diarrhea, Studentlitteratur, 1986, Lund.

Lebenthal, E., and Duffey, M.E., editors: Textbook of secretory diarrhea, Raven Press, Inc., 1990, New York.

Lewis, G.E., Jr., editor: Viral hepatitis: biological and clinical features, Raven Press, Inc., 1991, New York.

Meyer, E.A., editor: Giardiasis, Elsevier Science Publishers B.V., 1990, Amsterdam.

Smith, L.D.S., and Sugiyama, H.: Botulism: the organism, its toxins, the disease, C.C. Thomas, 1988, Springfield.

Tzipori, S.: Infectious diarrhea in the young, Elsevier Medical Pub., 1985, Amsterdam.

Case 1 The Church Picnic

Betty B. was exhausted after the volleyball tournament, held as part of the annual August church picnic. After that vigorous exercise, she had three glasses of lemonade and stuffed herself from the large picnic table laden with ham salad sandwiches, potato chips, three-bean salad, fresh sliced tomatoes, and chocolate cake. When evening came, Betty prepared herself for an early bedtime. Although it was only 9:15, she felt tired and a little feverish, which she attributed to a slight sunburn.

At 11 PM, she awoke sharply with stomach pain and an urge to vomit. She broke out in a cold sweat as she vomited into the toilet bowl. Her stomach cramps were slightly relieved as she delivered a loose bowel movement. Although she felt extremely nauseous and had the death wish typical of severe diarrhea, she survived several episodes of vomiting, intestinal cramps, and further loose stools. By 4 o'clock, she was able to fall asleep and slept for the remainder of the night.

At breakfast time, she felt weak, was decidedly thirsty, but had a good appetite, ate well, and felt well enough to leave for work. She wondered if any of her friends at the picnic spent the night as she had.

Questions

1. What is meant by the term *food poisoning*?
2. Do Betty's symptoms suggest a food intoxication or a food infection?
3. What foods available at the church picnic are the most likely source of Betty's illness?
4. What growth characteristics of bacteria are compatible with your answer to question 3?
5. Would you eliminate a viral etiology of this case?
6. What microbiologic procedures would you choose to identify the etiology of this case?
7. Is bacteriophage typing useful here?
8. What is an enterotoxin?
9. Can an exotoxin be an enterotoxin?
10. Do you suspect that others in attendance at the picnic suffered the same experience as Betty?
11. Will Betty be immune to another attack of food poisoning by the same agent?
12. How does food become "poisoned" in cases like this?

Student Questions

Case 2 A Barrio in Lima

José Carillo and his family were battling to survive in the Chiclayo barrio of Lima, Peru. Their shelter consisted of a rough framework covered with scraps of lumber, sheet metal, canvas, and cardboard. They had no running water, no gas, and no toilet or bathing facilities, and their floor was hard-packed earth. The children cleansed themselves by washing or swimming at the nearby ocean shore. Fields near their home were used as toilets. Water was collected for family use in cooking and drinking from a small spring that surfaced near the roadway that separated the field from the ocean beach.

José was unemployed and had a meager income from items he could salvage from a nearby dump heap and sell. The family poverty caused the children to beg for food and money. On January 28, 1991, Raul, age 6, the youngest son of the Carillo family, began to have diarrhea. Several loose stools were delivered that day. Raul did not complain of intestinal cramps and did not vomit. His family believed that this would go away quickly, since they had experienced diarrhea in the family many times. But this was not realized when Raul continued to have bouts of diarrhea during the night. By midday of January 29, Raul was taken to the Social Security Medical Clinic by his mother. When seen by a physician, Raul explained that he had been wading and washing himself almost daily at the ocean edge. He had eaten beans and rice at home but had found a partially eaten cheese sandwich in a waste can at the ocean shore some days earlier (he wasn't certain when) and had eaten it. He had consumed no milk for several weeks.

Questions

1. With this socioeconomic history, is there any evidence to suggest one etiology over another for this case?
2. Given the knowledge of a cholera epidemic in Peru in 1991, could this be cholera?
3. How can cholera be distinguished from other toxic forms of gastroenteritis?
4. What is the most likely source of the infection?
5. By what method does the cholera bacillus cause gastroenteritis?
6. How does your answer to question 5 differ if asked for *Escherichia coli* rather than the cholera vibrio?
7. What are the bacteriologic characteristics of *Vibrio cholerae*?
8. Are there special growth conditions of the cholera bacillus compared to other gram-negative bacteria?
9. Does a bout of cholera provide good long-term immunity?
10. What is the status of cholera vaccines?
11. Is there any reason to eliminate a virus as the etiologic agent of this disease?
12. What animal parasites could account for Raul's diarrhea?
13. What therapy is recommended for cholera?
14. What is the biochemical (physiologic) basis for the diarrhea in cholera?
15. How would knowledge of other cases of diarrhea in Raul's barrio influence your evaluation of the etiology of his diarrhea?

Student Questions

Case 3 The Love Boat

Captain Seifert was raging. Seventy-five people had flooded the ship's medical office the second morning at sea, and now it was apparent that as many as 50% of the cruise passengers had diarrhea. Captain Seifert had radioed for medical assistance, and a team of three physicians from the Centers for Disease Control would soon board the ship. Captain Seifert already knew what the medical experts would learn—exactly the same things they learned from the previous cruise.

On the previous sailing, eventually 60% of the passengers developed diarrhea. Most of the victims became ill within 24 hours after their first shipboard meal. Some thought at first that their vomiting was just a touch of seasickness, but when their nausea extended to abdominal cramps, diarrhea, sweats, and chills (some even had muscle pain), they realized it was something else. Soon the sheer number of sick individuals made it clear that help was needed, as it was once again today. Hopefully, the medical experts would have better success determining the cause of this episode than they did last time.

Questions

1. What etiologic agents are associated with massive outbreaks of diarrhea?
2. What bacterial agent is most responsible for acute gastroenteritis on a worldwide basis?
3. What viral agents are potential sources of this outbreak?
4. How is the viral etiology of acute gastroenteritis determined?
5. Would you expect to find an index case of diarrhea among the passengers?
6. Would you expect to find an index case of diarrhea among the crew?
7. Which crew members are most prone to develop diarrhea acquired from the passengers?
8. What foods are involved in viral diarrheas?
9. Is this second outbreak related to the earlier cruise experience?

10. Are future cruises at hazard for recurrences of acute gastroenteritis of the same etiology?
11. What is the therapy for viral gastroenteritis?
12. What is the morbidity and mortality of viral gastroenteritis?

Student Questions

Case 4 A Sickening Meal

John's seminar had gone very well, very well indeed. He'd had a lot of questions leveled at him, most of which he had thought of before. The few new questions were a little tougher, especially those from members of the search committee, but he thought he'd handled them with aplomb. Later, as his interview continued in the department chairman's office, he was gratified to learn that the job was his if he so chose. He could start in July as an assistant professor of history.

That evening John, the members of the search committee, and several other faculty members met at the chairman's home for cocktails. The snacks consisted of the usual selection of crackers, an especially delicious swiss cheese, chips, and both guacamole and an onion–sour cream dip. Everyone seemed to eat heavily from the snack trays—at least the food was pretty well gone when the group disbanded.

The search committee and the chairman had arranged for dinner at the Peking Garden Restaurant, so this portion of the group reconvened at 8 PM. As is customary, everyone ordered a different dish, which they shared with the others along with generous portions of both boiled and fried rice. Unfortunately the meal had hardly begun when Maxine, a member of the search committee, was called to the phone. With apologies, she excused herself from the dinner to go home and solve her babysitter's problem.

The Chinese banquet continued, and the fortune cookies weren't brought to the table until nearly 11 PM. John was dropped off at the hotel with the understanding that the chairman would meet him there at 8:30 in the morning for breakfast. Last-minute concerns could be discussed before John took the airport limousine for his 11 AM departure.

At 7:30 the next morning, the chairman received a call from John asking that they cancel the breakfast. John had been ill since about 3 or 4 in the morning. He had vomited several times, had only one loose stool, but was obviously concerned about getting through the breakfast without a lot of inconvenience and embarrassment. When the chairman related that he had almost exactly the same experience during the night and had been advised by his physician that he would probably feel completely well again by noon, John refused the chairman's offer of a physician's services and went back to bed. As expected, he felt well enough to eat a small lunch and was able to reschedule his flight home for 6:15 that evening.

Questions

1. Which is the most likely source of this gastroenteritis—the cocktail party or the Chinese dinner? Why?
2. Which foods do you think are most probably incriminated?
3. Does the incubation time suggest a viral disease, an intoxication, or an infection?
4. Would you expect all persons, including Maxine, to have this illness?
5. Discuss immunity to food poisoning relative to your answer to question 4.
6. What is the mode of action of enterotoxins? Do they all behave in the same way?
7. How do viruses cause diarrhea?
8. Discuss the heat stability of specific enterotoxins.
9. How do bacteria and enterotoxins survive in the digestive system?
10. How are diarrheas of viral origin diagnosed?

Student Questions

Case 5 Captain Courageous

Douglas Anacker, a 37-year-old pilot for an international airline company, took advantage of his profession to enjoy a 1-week ski vacation in Northern Italy. The ski resort was in an isolated area not yet frequented by the international crowd. The resort had its own water purification and sewage disposal system. The food was excellent, and the wines were well chosen. After his vacation, Doug returned to Milan to relax for 2 short days before resuming his position as captain on the Milan–New York flight. On the morning of his flight, Doug had a gaseous, explosive bowel movement, but since he didn't feel particularly ill, he thought this was just an incidental bowel complaint. Doug decided to report for his flight, which left on schedule for New York.

En route Captain Anacker's condition worsened. He had numerous loose stools, abdominal distention, feelings of nausea, and cramping. Finally he had to give command of the aircraft to the copilot. Upon arrival in New York, Captain Anacker reported to the airline medical officer, who noted the captain had a fever and was severely dehydrated. The doctor made note of the time Captain Anacker had spent on vacation and in Milan. He decided to examine a stool specimen for ova and parasites, from which he was able to establish the diagnosis and prescribe treatment.

Questions

1. Isn't a stool examination for ova and parasites routine in cases of diarrhea?
2. How is a stool specimen treated to recover ova or parasites?
3. Describe the life cycle of parasites associated with diarrhea.
4. What is the expected resistance of viruses, bacteria, ova, and cysts to water purification methods?
5. Is it possible to determine the incubation time of this diarrhea? What are the possibilities?
6. What is the role of the normal gut flora in preventing diarrheas?
7. What medication would you recommend for Captain Anacker?
8. Discuss the use of oral rehydration salts in treating diarrheas.

Student Questions

Case 6 Day Care and Weekend Care

Toddler Care, the city government–sponsored day care center in the Southside tenement area, normally cared for 73 children every day. Preschool children from age 1 to 5 were eligible to enroll, but practically all the children were between 1 and 3. All were from low-income families representing several minorities, with blacks and Hispanics being the dominant groups.

On Friday of last week, two of the children had a sudden onset of watery diarrhea at 3 PM. The nurse examined both children and found that they had a definite fever (101°F and 101.5°F) and the expected symptoms of lower abdominal cramping, tenderness, and signs of toxemia. When the children's mothers called for them after work, the nurse cautioned both parents about the status of their children and advised them to observe the children for continued diarrhea and seek medical attention if necessary. She emphasized the need to force fluids on the children. She stressed the importance of personal hygiene in preventing the spread of the disease to other family members.

Toddler Care was closed over the weekend. On Monday, the attendance was down to 57. Several mothers called in to report that their children had diarrhea. During the week, the attendance fell to 37 on Thursday but was up to 53 on Friday. Some children who were absent earlier returned on Thursday, and even more returned on Friday. By the following Monday, the attendance had returned to its normal level. One child was absent with chickenpox, and two had been hospitalized because of their serious diarrhea. Both mothers of the hospitalized children called in to say their children had a bacterial diarrhea.

Questions

1. Which are the contagious and which are the noncontagious forms of diarrheas?
2. Which species of bacteria cause most diarrheas in child care centers?
3. How is the diagnosis of bacterial diarrhea usually made in the laboratory?
4. Is a Gram stain of a stool specimen ever defensible?
5. What enrichment media are used in enteric microbiology?
6. Discuss the composition of plating media used in enteric microbiology.
7. How are nonsecretory bacterial diarrheas treated?
8. What other circumstances may lead to child and adult epidemics of diarrhea?
9. What is the role of carriers in bacterial diarrheas?
10. Which bacterial diarrhea(s) can be considered a zoonotic disease?
11. What is your prediction about the effect of the case of chickenpox on the Toddler Care center?
12. Describe the etiologic agent of chickenpox.
13. Couldn't this situation be cryptosporidiosis, giardiasis, or other parasitic disease?

Student Questions

Case 7 The Ice Cream Party

The annual ice cream party for the kindergarten class at Fulton Grade School was held on the last day of school, a Thursday. Ice cream had been made in the school's kitchen using their standard recipe—vanilla, pasteurized milk and cream, eggs, and sugar. The ice cream had been served to the children with their choice of chocolate or butterscotch syrup. Chocolate brownies and peanut crunch cookies were also available. All of the ice cream was devoured by the children. The leftover brownies and cookies were taken home by the volunteer parents who had donated them. Remains of the syrup were still in the school's refrigerators on Monday and when tested proved to be free of pathogenic bacteria.

These historical data are of interest because between Friday morning and Monday morning 17 of the 20 children in the class developed fever, some as high as 104.2°F, diarrhea, and abdominal cramps. Most of the affected children also had headaches, muscle aches, and vomiting. Three of the children had bloody stools.

Since none of the food was available for microbiologic analysis and no adults had become ill, it was not possible to prove the source or identity of the food responsible for this outbreak, but it was concluded that the ice cream was the most likely source.

Questions

1. Isn't it rare to consider ice cream as a source of food poisoning?
2. Does the presence of a bloody stool suggest any particular pathogenic group(s)?
3. What is the role of urinalysis in the bacteriologic diagnosis of diarrhea?
4. What is the role of blood cultures in the diagnosis of diarrhea?
5. Where do serologic tests fit into the diagnosis of diarrheas of undetermined origin?
6. Describe the chemistry of the O antigen of the enterobacteria.
7. What procedures are used to isolate pathogens from frozen foods?

8. Other than rehydration, what therapy is advised for these children?
9. What is the prospect that some of the parents will become ill?
10. Describe prophylactic therapy against diarrheal diseases.

Student Questions

Case 8 Get Hep

Selmon, a 39-year-old cook employed at the City Diner Restaurant, was surprised when he saw the uniformed man enter the kitchen. It didn't matter anyway—he'd been off drugs for 3 months and could claim he didn't know the latest neighborhood pushers. But the visitor wasn't a police officer; he was the supervisor of the city health officer who dropped in unexpectedly for inspection every 2 or 3 weeks.

The supervisor told Selmon that an outbreak of hepatitis infection had erupted in the city. Most of the hepatitis patients lived in this part of the city, and several had been regular customers for lunch here at the diner. Food handlers at this, among several restaurants on this side of town, were being examined as potential carriers of hepatitis virus.

Questions

1. How is hepatitis transmitted? Is this the same for hepatitis A, hepatitis B, and the non-A non-B forms of hepatitis?
2. Describe the hepatitis A virus, including its replicative cycle.
3. How are hepatitis A virus carriers detected?
4. How are hepatitis B virus carriers detected?
5. Is there a vaccine against hepatitis?
6. What postexposure prophylaxis is available for hepatitis?
7. When the source of hepatitis infections is removed, does that mean no more cases will appear? What is the incubation period of hepatitis?
8. What are common vehicles of hepatitis A and B transmission?
9. What is Australia antigen? Does it fit into this case?
10. What, if any, is the possibility of hepatitis C, D (the delta agent), or E being involved in this case?

Student Questions

Review Questions

1. Which of the following enteric pathogens does **not** invade intestinal epithelial cells?
   A. *Campylobacter jejuni*
   B. *Salmonella typhimurium*
   C. *Shigella dysenteriae* type 1
   D. *Vibrio cholerae*
   E. *Yersinia enterocolitica*

2. Which of the following tests would be most useful to differentiate *Shigella flexneri* from *Shigella boydii*?
   A. Agglutination in specific antisera
   B. Fermentation of lactose
   C. Motility
   D. Production of H_2S
   E. Triple sugar iron (TSI) agar reactions

3. The LT (heat-labile toxin) of enterotoxigenic *Escherichia coli* (ETEC) is
   A. Actually its LPS (lipopolysaccharide)
   B. Structurally identical in all known respects to exotoxin A from *Pseudomonas aeruginosa*
   C. Of low molecular weight, below the threshold of antigenicity
   D. Composed of 5 B units and 5 A units
   E. Toxic by the same biochemical-physiologic process as that of toxigenic *Vibrio cholerae*

4. Which of the following diseases is **not** caused by an exotoxin composed of a binding unit and an enzyme unit?
   A. Cholera
   B. Scarlet fever

C. Diphtheria
D. Pertussis
E. Diarrhea due to enterotoxic *E. coli*

5. Which of the following is **not** true of *E. coli*?

A. It is a facultative inhabitant of the large intestine.
B. It is usually nonmotile and is unable to ferment lactose.
C. It is a common cause of urinary tract infections.
D. It is classified by its O, H, and K antigens.
E. It is the most common etiology of traveler's diarrhea.

6. Which of the following water-borne agents is most resistant to chlorination?

A. *Escherichia coli*
B. *Giardia lamblia*
C. *Shigella boydii*
D. *Campylobacter jejuni*
E. *Salmonella typhi*

7. *Salmonella* species

A. Can be considered as zoonotic pathogens
B. Are transmitted to man from contaminated food and water
C. Produce colorless colonies on SS agar
D. Are serogrouped on the basis of their O antigens
E. All of the above

8. Which of the following produces a heat-stable enterotoxin?

A. *Clostridium botulinum*
B. *Staphylococcus aureus*
C. *Salmonella typhi*
D. *Shigella dysenteriae*
E. *Shigella boydii*

9. Adherence factors are very important for which one of the following agents of gastroenteritis?

A. *Clostridium botulinum*
B. *Bacillus cereus*
C. *Entamoeba histolytica*
D. *Staphylococcus aureus*
E. *Vibrio cholerae*

10. Viral gastroenteritis is most often associated with which of the following list?

A. Reoviruses
B. Orthomyxoviruses
C. Herpes viruses
D. Picornaviruses
E. Arboviruses

11. Which of the following agents of gastroenteritis is associated with a short incubation time of the disease it produces?

A. *Vibrio cholerae*
B. *Escherichia coli*
C. *Staphylococcus aureus*
D. *Salmonella typhimurium*
E. *Giardia lamblia*

12. Which of the following produces a yellow slant, yellow butt, and gas on growth in a TSI slant?

A. *Vibrio cholerae*
B. *Escherichia coli*
C. *Staphylococcus aureus*
D. *Salmonella typhimurium*
E. *Giardia lamblia*

13. *Clostridium botulinum*

A. Can be distinguished from other clostridia by its formation of terminal endospores
B. Spores in honey are a source of infant botulism
C. Toxins are formed abundantly by growth of the organism in canned, acidic foods
D. Toxin acts on the neuromuscular synapse
E. Exists in two antigenic types

14. Antibiotic-associated colitis has been linked to a toxin produced by which one of the following organisms?

A. *Clostridium perfringens*
B. *Bacteroides fragilis*
C. *Bacteroides melaninogenicus*
D. *Clostridium difficile*
E. *Campylobacter fetus*

15. The following are characteristics of the exotoxin (neurotoxin) of *Clostridium botulinum* **except**

A. May be produced in the intestinal tract of infants colonized with spores
B. Can be neutralized by antitoxin after the toxin is fixed to cells
C. Produces a flaccid muscle paralysis
D. Exists in several different serologic types
E. may be destroyed by boiling for 10 minutes or longer

5 Genitourinary and Sexually Transmitted Diseases

There is a distinct overlap of infectious diseases of the genitourinary system and sexually transmitted diseases. Most conditions of the former group also fall into the latter category. Exceptions include urinary tract infections caused by gram-negative enteric bacteria and vaginitis in sexually inactive females caused by the yeast *Candida albicans*. Enteric bacteria can be mobilized by sexual activity, but cystitis of the sexually inactive female can also arise from these organisms as part of the fecal flora. *Candida* may be transmitted sexually, but many infants become colonized by this yeast during the birth process and retain the yeast as part of the normal intestinal or genitourinary flora thereafter.

Sexually transmitted diseases are frequently grouped according to the external symptoms of the disease, since these provide an excellent clue to their etiology. Ulcerative diseases include primary syphilis, chancroid, herpes, and the more rare granuloma inguinale. Diseases with a significant discharge reflect a colonization and inflammation of the mucosal surfaces and include gonorrhea, nongonococcal urethritis due to chlamydia and mycoplasma, and the female forms of trichomoniasis and vaginosis. Candidiasis may take many forms. The recent confirmation that genital neoplasms are induced by herpes virus, papillomavirus, and the agent of molluscum contagiosum adds another component to the spectrum of sexually transmitted diseases.

It is important to recognize that certain sexually transmitted diseases may cause little or no abnormality in genitourinary function. This is most clearly demonstrated in AIDS, but secondary or tertiary syphilis, asymptomatic *Trichomonas* infections in males, and asymptomatic gonorrhea in females are additional examples. Many sexually transmitted diseases may progress to serious conditions in other organ systems (e.g., neurosyphilis, AIDS dementia, pelvic inflammatory disease, arthritis), thus the importance of early and effective therapy.

The group of organisms causing sexually transmitted diseases is expansive and includes several varieties of bacteria, viruses, and at least one yeast and one animal parasite. Table 5-1 lists most of these organisms, their major characteristics, and important aspects of the diseases they cause.

Table 5-1. Common agents of genitourinary and sexually transmitted diseases*

Organism	Classification	Disease	Primary symptom	Secondary disease
Calymmatobacterium granulomatis	Bacterium	Lymphogranuloma inguinale	Papule, ulcer, and enlarged inguinal local lymph nodes (pseudobubos)	
Candida albicans	Yeast	Vaginitis	Yellow-green frothy discharge	
Chlamydia trachomatis	Bacterium	Nongonoccocal urethritis or lymphogranuloma venereum	Purulent urethritis, enlarged local lymph nodes (bubos)	Perirectal fissures
Escherichia coli and other enteric bacteria	Bacterium	Cystitis	Dysuria, lower back pain	
Gardnerella vaginalis	Gram-negative bacterium	Vaginosis	Foul-smelling discharge	
Haemophilus ducreyi	Gram-negative bacillus	Chancroid	Chancroid	
Hepatitis B	Virus	Hepatitis	Liver disease	Hepatocarcinoma
Herpes simplex 2 (or 1)	Virus	Herpes	Vesicles	Recurrent infections, cervical cancer
HIV virus	Retrovirus	AIDS	No genital symptoms	Immunodeficiency
Molluscum contagiosum	Poxvirus		Benign skin lesion	
Mycoplasma hominis	Mycoplasma	Nongonococcal urethritis	Purulent urethritis	
Neisseria gonorrhoeae	Gram-negative coccus	Gonorrhea	Purulent urethritis	Gonococcal arthritis, pelvic inflammatory disease
Papillomavirus	Virus	Condyloma acuminatum	Genital warts	Cervical cancer
Treponema pallidum	Spirochete	Syphilis	Painless ulcer (chancre)	Congenital and advanced forms of syphilis
Trichomonas vaginalis	Flagellate protozoan	Vaginitis	Foamy discharge	
Ureaplasma urealyticum	Mycoplasma	Nongonococcal urethritis	Purulent urethritis	

*Diseases due to ectoparasites are not included

Key Words and Phrases

These terms and abbreviations are part of the vocabulary you should master on completion of these problem cases.

Antigenemia
Australia antigen
Bacterial vaginosis
Bacteriuria
Bubo
Cardiolipin
Chancroid
Chlamydospores (chlamydoconidia)
Clue cells
Cold hemagglutinin test
Credé's prophylaxis
Cystitis
Dane particle
Darkfield microscopy
Dysuria
Elementary body
Gumma (gummatous lesions)
Hard chancre
Jarisch–Herxheimer reaction
Latent syphilis
Midstream catch
Ophthalmia neonatorum
Oxidase test
Primary syphilis
Pseudohyphae
Pyelonephritis
Reticulate body
Reverse transcriptase
Secondary syphilis
Soft chancre
Syphilitic reagin
Tertiary syphilis
Wassermann test

Abbreviations

AIDS
AZT
FTA–ABS
HBcAg
HBeAg
HBsAg
HBV
HIV
HSV
LGV
NGU
PID
PPNG
RPR
STD
TPI
UTI
VDRL

Information Sources

AIDS: information on AIDS for the practicing physician, American Medical Association, 1987, Chicago.

Bodey, G.P., editor: Candidiasis, edition 2, Raven Press, Inc., 1993, New York.

Brooks, G.F., and Donegan, E.A.: Gonococcal infection, Edward Arnold, 1985, London.

Crum, C.P., and Nuovo, G.J.: Genital papillomaviruses and related neoplasms, Raven Press, 1991, New York.

Gallo, R.C., and Jay, G., editors: The human retroviruses, Academic Press, Inc., 1991, San Diego.

Gross, G., et al., editors: Genital papillomavirus infection, Springer-Verlag, 1990, Berlin.

Hamilton, G.C., et al.: Emergency medicine: an approach to clinical problem solving, W.B. Saunders Co., 1991, Philadelphia.

Holmes, K.K., et al.: Sexually transmitted diseases, edition 2, McGraw-Hill, 1990, New York.

Kunin, C.M.: Detection, prevention, and management of urinary tract infections, edition 4, Lea & Febiger, 1987, Philadelphia.

Leoung, G., and Mills, J., editors: Opportunistic infections in patients with acquired immunodeficiency syndrome, Marcel Dekker, Inc., 1989, New York.

Mardh, P.-A., Paavonen, J., and Puolakkainen, M.: Chlamydia, Plenum Medical Book Co., 1989, New York.

Morse, S.A., Moreland, A.A., and Thompson, S.E., editors: Atlas of sexually transmitted diseases, Raven Press, Inc., 1990, New York.

Olds, F.C.: *Candida* and the candidoses, W.B. Saunders Co., 1988, Philadelphia.

Parish, L.C., Sehgal, V.N., and Buntin, D.M.: Color atlas of sexually transmitted diseases, Igaku-Shoin Medical Publishers, Inc., 1991, New York.

Poolman, J.T., et al., editors: Gonococci and meningococci, Kluwer Academic Publishers, 1988, Dordrecht.

Quinn, T.C., editor: Sexually transmitted diseases, Raven Press, Inc., 1992, New York.

Remington, J.S., and Klein, J.O., editors: Infectious diseases of the fetus and newborn infant, edition 3, W.B. Saunders Co., 1990, Philadelphia.

Roberts, R.B., editor: The gonococci, John Wiley and Sons, 1977, New York.

Smith, D.M., Jr., and Dodd, R.Y., editors: Transfusion-transmitted infections, ASCP Press, 1991, Chicago.

Stamey, T.A.: Urinary infections, Williams & Wilkins Co., 1980, Baltimore.

Watstein, S.B., and Laurich, R.A.: AIDS and women: a sourcebook, Oryx Press, 1991, Phoenix.

Wood, M.J., and Farrar, W.E.: Atlas of genitourinary infections, Raven Press, Inc., 1992, New York.

Case 1 Honeymoon Hotel

Hannah, a 24-year-old newlywed, had spent 5 leisurely days at the island resort with her husband, Bill. She hadn't complained, but this hyperactive sex life was beginning to create a little discomfort. Last night it was a feeling that she hadn't completely emptied her bladder when urinating. Maybe the burning sensation had somehow caused her to hold it back. But when she tried to urinate again, a half hour later, she was still able to deliver only a few drops.

This morning it was even more uncomfortable, not just when urinating, but now she was beginning to notice some lower back pain. By noon her back pain was getting pretty uncomfortable so she called the hotel physician.

The hotel physician was very understanding. He said he'd seen this in a number of young newlyweds. He took Hannah's temperature (99.5°F) and asked her to collect some urine in a small plastic cup, but to wait until she was near the end of her delivery. Hannah was given a prescription for sulfamethoxazole-trimethoprim. The doctor left saying that he would call tomorrow to confirm his diagnosis and to see if she was feeling better. He cautioned Hannah to drink lots of water or other fluids while taking the medication.

Questions

1. How does a hyperactive sex life lead to genitourinary tract infections?
2. What are the usual routes of urinary tract infections?
3. What are the usual gram-negative bacteria involved in urinary tract infections?
4. What are the virulence properties of these bacteria?
5. What gram-positive organisms are the most frequently found in urinary tract diseases?
6. What is Bill's status regarding this infection—immune, immune carrier, susceptible, etc.?
7. How is the microbial diagnosis of this disease established?
8. What is chronic bacteriuria?
9. What factors predispose to cystitis?
10. Is the therapy appropriate in this case?
11. Some women have a chronic bacteriuria. How is this explained?
12. What bacterial adhesins contribute to urinary tract infections?

Student Questions

Case 2 Sick at Sea

A 21-year-old sailor, Ralph N., appeared at morning sick bay on the U.S.S. *Columbia* just 3 days at sea. Ralph told the hospital corpsman that he had a dose of clap. Ralph had intercourse with a prostitute in Bangkok the night before shipping out and blamed her for his infection. Yesterday he began to have painful urination (dysuria) and in the evening began to have a urethral discharge.

A cursory physical examination found no other symptoms of disease. Blood pressure, temperature, pulse rate, and respirations were all within the normal range. The urethral discharge was dominated by neutrophils, many of which contained gram-negative diplococci.

The navy doctor tentatively agreed with Ralph's original diagnosis and stated that although he was prescribing antibiotics, further tests would be needed to confirm the diagnosis and his present choice of antibiotics.

Questions

1. Why aren't gram-negative intracellular diplococci in a urethral discharge considered as positive proof of gonorrhea?
2. What tests provide positive identification of *Neisseria gonorrhoeae*?
3. What antibiotic do you think was prescribed?
4. What is the meaning of the abbreviation *PPNG*?
5. Is antibiotic resistance of gonococci a plasmid-mediated characteristic?
6. What are the complications of untreated or improperly treated gonorrhea?
7. Are these complications more severe in males or females?
8. What form does neonatal gonorrhea take? How is it treated or prevented?
9. How do gonococci establish their infection?
10. Explain why there is so little immunity to repeated gonococcal infections.
11. What is the status of vaccine development against gonorrhea?
12. What other sexually transmitted bacterial diseases are also possible in a patient with gonorrhea?
13. Do colony type differences of *N. gonorrhoeae* relate to virulence?
14. What are protein I and protein II of *N. gonorrhoeae*?
15. Does nonvenereal transmission of gonorrhea occur?

Student Questions

Case 3 Sexual Assault

Lois, a 23-year-old female graduate student, was brought to the emergency department at 2 AM by a volunteer woman from the local rape crisis center. Lois had been sexually assaulted in her apartment, where she lived alone. After recovering from the attack, she called the rape crisis center hotline.

Lois and the volunteer were escorted to a private area of the emergency department by a female physician, who carefully explained the necessity of certain procedures to establish that physical assault, including rape, had occurred.

Contusions on the neck, wrists, and near her left eye, which was swollen nearly closed, confirmed Lois's account of the physical attack. Swabs of vaginal secretions were examined microscopically and revealed the presence of spermatozoa. Lois was offerred treatment to prevent sexually transmitted diseases (STDs) after additional vaginal material and a blood culture were collected to determine if an STD was already present.

Lois spent the remainder of the night and the following 24 hours at the rape crisis center before returning to her apartment. Six days later she returned to the hospital to provide additional vaginal cultures. Six weeks later she returned to the hospital to give blood for repeat serologic tests.

Questions

1. Which STDs are usually diagnosed by direct examination of vaginal material?
2. Which diseases are diagnosed by culture?
3. Which STDs can be diagnosed by serologic tests?
4. What antibiotic treatment is best for victims of rape?
5. Why were vaginal cultures repeated after 1 week?
6. Describe serologic tests for syphilis.
7. Describe the status of immunity to STD.
8. Why is mucosal IgA generally unable to provide good immunity to STD?
9. Describe the stages of syphilis.
10. What is the risk for contracting an STD after rape?

Student Questions

Case 4 Another Case?

Jamal B., a 21-year-old truck driver for a city delivery agency, returned to the Venereal Disease Clinic of the Public Health Department. He had visited the clinic 1 week earlier and was diagnosed as having gonorrhea. This diagnosis was based on the presence of a heavy purulent urethral discharge containing intracellular gram-negative diplococci in polymorphonuclear leukocytes. Jamal had visited several different prostitutes prior to his first visit to the clinic, where he was treated with a penicillin.

The first 2 or 3 days after leaving the clinic his urethral discharge seemed to lighten, but now, 1 week later, he still had some slight drainage. Jamal had heard of penicillin-resistant gonorrhea and so returned to the VD clinic.

Jamal assured the Public Health physician that he had had no sexual contacts in the last week and that he wanted a stronger antibiotic to clear up his "clap."

Questions

1. What is the frequency of PPNG?
2. Is penicillin resistance of *Neisseria gonorrhoeae* a plasmid, phage, or chromosomally controlled event?
3. How does antigenic variation of the gonococcus occur—transformation, transduction, etc?
4. If this is a case of PPNG infection, what therapy would you choose now?
5. If this is not a case of PPNG infection, what are the other etiologic possibilities?
6. Describe the biochemistry of a cell wall–less microbe that could be responsible for this illness.
7. What is the metabolic target and mode of action of penicillin?
8. What antibiotics are effective in PPNG infections?
9. Shouldn't a patient with gonorrhea always be evaluated for other STDs?
10. What immunity can be expected to the agents of nongonococcal urethritis on recovery?
11. Was Jamal's earlier diagnosis of gonorrhea properly determined?

Student Questions

Case 5 A Problem at College

Sara, a sophomore college student, had moved into her apartment in September. It was a big change from last year's life in the dormitory and would have been a little lonely if it hadn't been for Steve.

She had met Steve in the organic chemistry class, where she had drawn him as a partner in laboratory. Steve was a sharp, handsome chemical engineering major. Within a month they were in love, and on the final weekend in October after the homecoming celebration, Steve stayed at Sara's apartment.

On Friday of the next week, Sara was at the student health clinic. She had an extreme amount of vaginal itching, dysuria, and a mild headache and felt a little feverish. The physician observed a mixture of vesiculopustular lesions and shallow, coalesced ulcers bilaterally present on the labia. Local edema was extensive. An internal gynecologic examination could not be made because of extreme discomfort as the speculum was inserted.

One of the outer lesions was scraped as gently as possible, and a microscopic smear was prepared. Acyclovir ointment was applied. Sara was told she would probably have recurrences of this condition and that she should avoid all sexual contact during the active stage of her disease and for 1 week thereafter.

Questions

1. How could Steve, in the absence of any obvious illness, transmit an STD to Sara?
2. Which STDs present as vesicular lesions?
3. Approximately how long will Sara have these lesions?
4. What is the mode of action of acyclovir?
5. What would be seen in the microscopic smear of the lesions?
6. Does this disease pass from person to person only by sexual contact?
7. Describe the basis of latency and recurrences of this disease.
8. How can the etiologic agent be isolated between episodes?
9. Many patients with this disease have high specific antibody titers. Explain this in relationship to protective immunity.
10. Compare this disease as it presents in males and females.

Student Questions

Case 6 The Hemophiliac

Phil A., a 52-year-old hemophiliac, had received blood transfusions and blood component (Factor VIII) therapy since 1962. He presented himself to his family physician with vague feelings of tiredness, shortness of breath, and occasional fever, which had developed over the past 4 or more weeks.

Physical examination revealed the following:

Pulse	109
Respirations	39
Blood pressure	134/78 mm Hg
Temperature	100.1°F

There was no detectable lymphadenopathy, hepatosplenomegaly, or unusual skin lesions. His knee joints were deformed from repeated bleeding into the joints as a result of the hemophilia.

Blood was collected for white cell counts, from which it was determined that he had a lymphopenia. Flow cytometry was ordered and determined that the $CD4^+$ cell count was 72 cells/mm^3. Urinalysis was not revealing.

When Phil returned to his physician 2 weeks later for consultation regarding these test results, he complained of a severe headache and muscle weakness on one side of his body (hemiparesis). He was given a CT scan and MRI, both of which revealed a small lesion in his left brain.

Phil was started on a sulfanilamide, folic acid, pentamidine, and acyclovir. The last was instituted because it was felt that Phil might have a herpes virus encephalitis. His condition improved slightly over the next few weeks, and MRI showed a partial resolution of the cerebral lesion.

About 4 months later, after periodic visits to his physician for treatment of thrush and prognostic examinations, Phil contracted pneumonia. Lung biopsy confirmed the presence of *Pneumocystis*. Phil was placed in a mechanical ventilator and given pentamidine intravenously for 14 days. Despite this treatment, his condition continued to deteriorate, and he expired within 12 days, less than 6 months after his original diagnosis.

Questions

1. What is the mode of action of pentamidine?
2. What is the mode of action of acyclovir?
3. Describe the morphology and growth characteristics of the agent of thrush.
4. Describe the nature of *Pneumocystis*, including its life cycle.
5. Describe the replication of retroviruses.
6. Is herpes virus infection a serious threat for patients like Phil? Explain.
7. Describe the technique of flow cytometry to detect and enumerate lymphocytes.
8. What are normal values of $CD4^+$ lymphocytes, and how are they reduced during this disease?

9. Why was folic acid administered with the sulfanilamide?
10. What other infectious diseases affect patients like Phil?

Student Questions

Case 7 Another Form of Vacationer's Disease

Dr. Vegas, hotel physician in Puerto Vallarta, was called by the desk clerk and advised that a woman in Room 116 wanted his assistance. After a brief discussion on the telephone, Dr. Vegas advised the woman to visit his clinic only a few blocks from her hotel.

When Dr. Vegas met the woman in his clinic, he found her to be a typical female vacationer—young, tan, healthy, and well groomed. She repeated to him the same complaint she had voiced on the telephone. She had considerable vaginal irritation and had noticed a yellow staining of her underpants. She admitted to sexual intimacy with a new companion she had met since starting her vacation. Although he had no symptoms of disease and wished to continue their sexual relationship, she had too much discomfort to participate in sex.

Because of her evident general good health and focused symptoms, Dr. Vegas was already quite certain of the diagnosis. He made a cursory gynecologic examination, noting the heavy, frothy, yellow discharge and the classic strawberry cervix. Unfortunately, he could not confirm the diagnosis by a microscopic examination of the discharge but gave her a prescription and told her she would be much better in a day or two. Dr. Vegas cautioned her to be aware of other sexually transmitted diseases and to call him if she wasn't better within 2 days. He also asked for her male companion to take the medication as well.

Questions

1. What is the most probable etiologic agent of this disease?
2. What are the symptoms of this disease in males?
3. What is the cause of the pathognomonic strawberry cervix?

4. What is the female-male relationship in regard to the maintenance of this infection?
5. Does the etiologic agent have a resistant stage in its life cycle?
6. Is female-to-female transmission of this disease via fomites possible?
7. What type of microscopic examination normally identifies the etiologic agent?
8. Can this pathogen be cultivated?
9. What is the recommended therapy?
10. If the acute vaginitis subsided without treatment, would the woman become a carrier?

Student Questions

Review Questions

1. The following genera contain species that cause sexually transmitted disease except

   A. *Chlamydia*
   B. *Haemophilus*
   C. *Neisseria*
   D. *Rickettsia*
   E. *Treponema*

2. A male patient with culture-positive gonococcal urethritis was treated with prescribed doses of penicillin. A week later, he returned complaining of painful urination and a urethral discharge. Which of the following could be true?

   A. The patient may have become reinfected.
   B. He may have nongonococcal urethritis.
   C. The infection could be caused by a penicillinase-producing *Neisseria gonorrhoeae.*
   D. His wife may be asymptomatically infected with gonococci.
   E. All of the above are true.

3. *Neisseria gonorrhoeae* that possess pili (fimbriae)

A. Are virulent and produce disease
B. Produce different colony morphologies when compared to gonococci that have no pili
C. Can attach to cells of mucous membranes
D. Become avirulent if the cells lose the pili
E. All of the above

4. *Neisseria gonorrhoeae* can be distinguished from *Neisseria meningitidis* by

A. The oxidase test
B. Fermentation of glucose but not maltose
C. By its presence inside polymorphonuclear neutrophils
D. Its production of beta lactamase
E. None of the above

5. *Treponema pallidum*

A. Is the only pathogen in its genus
B. Infection is best diagnosed by serologic tests in the primary stages of the disease
C. Immobilization tests are the most commonly used diagnostic aid for primary syphilis
D. Infection is determined by a nonspecific antigen in the RPR test
E. Causes a lesion called the soft chancre

6. *Chlamydia trachomatis*

A. Has peptidoglycan
B. Contains sterols in its cytoplasmic membrane
C. Has a complex life cycle involving elementary and reticulate bodies
D. Causes only ocular infections
E. Infections are treatable with penicillin

7. Which of the following is true of AIDS?

A. The T_H/T_S cell ratio gradually increases.
B. The disease has an extended incubation period.
C. Azidothymidine (AZT) will cure AIDS.
D. The disease is produced only in persons with a previous immunocompromised condition.
E. Its etiologic agent is a DNA virus.

8. *Candida albicans* grows in vivo as

A. A mixture of yeast cells and pseudohyphae
B. Pure culture of yeast cells
C. Pure culture of pseudohyphae
D. An encapsulated yeast
E. Hyphae bearing chlamydospores

9. Vaginitis may be caused by

A. *Candida albicans*
B. *Trichomonas vaginalis*
C. *Gardnerella vaginalis*
D. Only B and C
E. A, B, and C

10. Which of these sexually transmitted agents is most frequently encountered as an asymptomatic infection in the United States?

A. *Treponema pallidum*
B. *Entamoeba histolytica*
C. *Chlamydia trachomatis*
D. *Candida albicans*
E. *Trichomonas vaginalis*

11. An important early step in the pathogenesis of *Escherichia coli* urinary tract infections is

A. Adherence to epithelial cells
B. Growth in the urine
C. Production of urease
D. Resistance to antibiotics
E. All of the above

12. The most common cause of urinary tract infections is

A. *Proteus vulgaris*
B. *Pseudomonas aeruginosa*
C. *Escherichia coli*
D. Due to enterococci
E. *Staphylococcus aureus*

13. A KOH wet mount of a specimen from a woman with vulvovaginitis reveals budding yeasts and hypha-like cell arrangements. Which of the following is most true?

A. The patient has a dual mycotic infection due to a yeast and a mold.
B. If the infection is due to a single agent, it should produce chlamydospores on Sabouraud's agar.
C. An India ink preparation would have been superior to the KOH wet mount for examination of the specimen.
D. The fungus is *Cryptococcus neoformans.*
E. Both C and D are true.

14. The Dane particle

A. Is the capsid of hepatitis A virus
B. Is the entire hepatitis A virion
C. Is related to the Australia antigen
D. Was discovered in Denmark
E. Is a common structure of all hepatitis viruses

15. Pelvic inflammatory disease of females is caused most often by

A. *Treponema pallidum*
B. *Candida albicans*
C. HIV
D. *Trichomonas vaginalis*
E. *Neisseria gonorrhoeae*

6 Skin and Wound Infections

The skin provides a formidable barrier against most microbes, and it is unlikely that pathogens can penetrate intact skin. Possible exceptions include a few sexually transmitted agents (*Treponema pallidum, Haemophilus ducreyi*) and the tularemia bacillus (*Francisella tularensis*). Even here, microscopic abrasions may provide the portal of entry. Some fungi may penetrate the hair follicles to initiate infections of the hair or skin.

The skin is often a window for the diagnosis of many airborne pathogens such as measles, chickenpox, meningococcal, streptococcal, and staphylococcal infections. The last two bacteria produce classic skin diseases—scarlet fever and scalded skin syndrome—yet the organisms are not present in the skin during these infections. These airborne conditions could be included here, since these diseases are expressed and diagnosed on the basis of changes in the skin.

The primary skin pathogens are restricted to the dermatophytic fungi, a few animal parasites, and several bacteria including the highly important staphylococci and streptococci. *Staphylococcus aureus* is associated with several types of skin abscesses including boils, carbuncles, furuncles, and folliculitis, the last of which is relatively minor but which may be slightly disfiguring. Impetigo, erysipelas, and cellulitis are most often caused by streptococci and staphylococci, sometimes in a mixed infection.

The approach to skin infections must first consider the acute or chronic nature of the disease. Fungal and mycobacterial infections are slowly progressing, mildly inflammatory diseases that patients often tolerate for several days, frequently with efforts at self-medication, before seeking medical attention. The fungal infections may involve the nail bed and the hair, areas not involved in mycobacterial infections. Whenever hot, highly inflamed vesicles or pustules form in the skin, a bacterial illness of an acute nature is usually the cause, and early medical attention is imperative (Table 6-1). Viral diseases may present as vesicular or pustular eruptions, or as erythematous rashes, depending on the etiology.

d Phrases

the terms related to the problem cases in this chapter relate to fungal patho- emember that these listings cannot be all-inclusive, and you may need to add o this list.

ype toxin
ylate cyclase
rospore
tospore
Cellulitis
Chlamydospore
Cigar body
Conidiophore
Dermatomycosis
Dimorphic fungus
Edema factor
Erysipelas
Erysipeloid
Eschar
Folliculitis
Herpetic whitlow
H-L type toxin
Lethal factor
Macroconidium
Malignant pustule
Microconidium
Mycetoma
Negri body
Onychomycosis
Protective antigen
Pseudohypha
Ringworm
Sabouraud's medium
Tetanospasmin
Varicella
Zoonosis

Abbreviations

EF
HSV
LF
PA
VZV

Information Sources

Aly, R., and Maibach, H.I.: Clinical skin microbiology, C.C. Thomas, 1978, Springfield.

Bodey, G.P., editor: Candidiasis, edition 2, Raven Press, Inc., 1993, New York.

duVivier, A.: Atlas of clinical dermatology, W.B. Saunders Co., 1986, Philadelphia.

duVivier, A.: Atlas of infections of the skin, Gowed Medical Publishing, 1991, London.

Finegold, S.M., Baron, E.J., and Wexler, H.M.: A clinical guide to anaerobe infections, Star Publishing Co., 1992, Belmont, CA.

Finegold, S.M., and George, W.L., editors: Anaerobic infections in humans, Academic Press, Inc., 1989, San Diego.

Table 6-1. Agents associated with skin and wound infections*

Agent		Disease
Ancylostoma brazcliense	Helminth	Cutaneous larva migrans
Ancylostoma duodenale	Helminth	Hookworm
Bacillus anthracis	Bacterium	Anthrax
Blastomyces dermatitidis	Fungus	Blastomycosis
Candida albicans	Yeast	Intertrigo, onychomycosis
Clostridium perfringens	Bacterium	Gas gangrene
Clostridium tetani	Bacterium	Tetanus
Epidermophyton floccosum	Fungi	Infections of skin, hair, and nails (ringworm)
Erysipelothrix rhusiopathiae	Bacterium	Erysipeloid
Francisella tularensis	Bacterium	Tularemia
Herpes simplex virus	Virus	Cold sores, fever blisters
Microsporum species	Fungus	Dermatophytic infection
Mycobacterium species	Bacteria	Skin ulcers, granuloma
Necator americanus	Helminth	Hookworm
Papilloma viruses	Virus	Warts
Pseudomonas aeruginosa	Bacterium	Hot-tub folliculitis
Pasteurella multocida	Bacterium	Cat-scratch fever
Sporothrix schenckii	Fungus	Sporotrichosis
Staphylococcus aureus	Bacterium	Folliculitis, carbuncles, etc.
Streptococcus pyogenes	Bacterium	Impetigo, erysipelas, etc.
Trichophyton species	Fungus	Dermatophytic infection
Varicella-zoster virus	Virus	Chickenpox, herpes zoster

*Does not include sexually transmitted diseases.

Habif, T.P.: Clinical dermatology: a color guide to diagnosis and therapy, C.V. Mosby Co., 1990, St. Louis.

Kwon-Chung, K.J., and Bennett, J.E.: Medical mycology, Lea & Febiger, 1992, Malvern, PA.

Laroner, D.H.: Medically important fungi, edition 2, ASM Press, 1993, Herndon, VA.

Maibach, H.I., and Aly, R., editors: Skin microbiology: relevance to clinical infection, Springer-Verlag, 1981, New York.

Moschella, S.L., and Hurley, H.J., editors: Dermatology, W.B. Saunders Co., 1985, Philadelphia.

Noble, W.C., editor: The skin microflora and microbial skin disease, Cambridge University Press, 1993, Cambridge.

Rook, A.J., and Maibach, H.I., editors: Recent advances in dermatology, Churchill Livingstone, 1983, Edinburgh.

Simpson, L.L., editor: Botulinum neurotoxin and tetanus toxin, Academic Press, Inc., 1989, San Diego.

Whitford, H.W.: A guide to the diagnosis, treatment, and prevention of anthrax, WHO, 1987, Geneva.

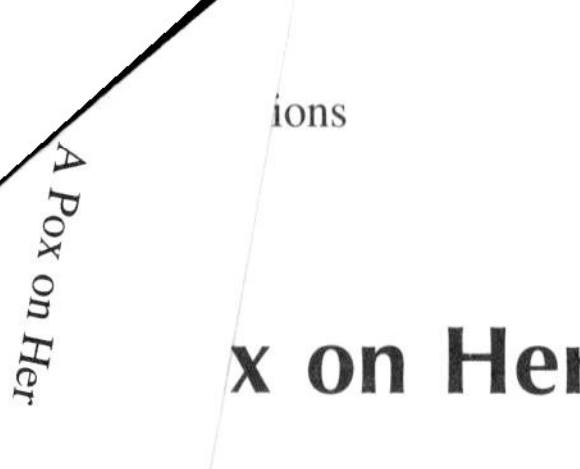

x on Her

, a 62-year-old housewife, called her physician because of increasing pain in t side at the intracostal juncture. She first noticed the pain 2 days ago. When eptionist said that all appointments were filled that day, Alice agreed to come office early the next morning rather than declare herself an emergency case. ring the night, the pain, though localized in a band across her body, became more severe. Aspirin did little to relieve it. In the morning, the pained area was med, and her skin in that region began to develop numerous small vesicles.

lice's physician was quite certain of the diagnosis and prescribed acyclovir. A cursory physical examination revealed no other condition or complaint other than a mild psoriasis that had affected Alice for the past 20 or more years.

The next day Alice's doctor conferred with her on the telephone. Alice described her affected area as extremely painful and covered with many blisters. Her doctor asked her to be certain to continue her medication for the next 2 weeks and to call him if the blisters changed their appearance, other than drying or other obvious signs of healing.

Four days later Alice called in to say that some of the blisters looked milky white and that one or two of these had broken open and had drained a few droplets of pus. Her physician asked Alice to report to his clinic immediately.

Questions

1. Is this an example of a primary, secondary, or latent infection?
2. Is a 62-year-old woman (partially) immunodeficient?
3. Why is this infection localized?
4. Does psoriasis predispose to this infection?
5. What is the mode of action of acyclovir?
6. Is it characteristic for these vesicles to become pustulent?
7. Why did her physician call her to the clinic immediately when pustules developed?
8. What skin diseases are characterized by painful vesicles?
9. Is there an effective vaccine against this disease in any of its stages?
10. Describe the etiologic agent in chemicophysical terms.
11. How is this disease acquired (transmitted)?
12. Name and describe agents closely related to the agent causing this disease.
13. What are the laboratory tests needed to confirm the diagnosis?
14. How have PCR studies contributed to our understanding of the life history of this agent?

Student Questions

Case 2 A Problem to Wrestle With

The wrestling team would have to withdraw from the finals. There was simply no way they could compete. Dick was the only team member who had escaped the skin disorder, whatever it was.

The team had checked into the city's leading hotel and after unpacking had gone to the gym for the opening round of competition on Thursday evening. Nothing especially eventful occurred during or after the match. None of their opponents had a noticeable skin disease. All team members showered, dressed, and returned to the hotel, except for Dick. Dick had permission to stay with his parents, who lived in the town where the tournament was being held.

At the hotel some of the aches and pains from the afternoon's competition were relieved in the hot tub in the hotel's health club facility.

The events Friday followed closely those of Thursday. Most members of the team had won their match in the round-robin competition and relaxed in the hot tub again before dinner. A couple of the guys, Frank and John, went swimming instead of to the hot tub.

Saturday afternoon, Dick found himself all alone at the gym where the tournament was being held. When he called the hotel, he learned that all six of his teammates had some kind of skin rash. Frank and John had an itching, raised, lumpy type of rash that didn't seem as bad as the others. Most of them had tiny blister-like eruptions that itched. Two other members had earaches, and two others had a sore throat. For athletes in good physical condition, all of them felt some tiredness or weakness.

The wrestling team coach reported all this to the hotel physician and the physicians assigned to the tournament. The hotel management decided to close the health club pending further information from the city sanitation officer about what they should do.

Questions

1. Why did Frank and John have a milder illness?
2. How did Dick escape the disease?
3. Do the cases of sore throat and ear infection suggest a respiratory route of infection?
4. What is the relationship of throat and ear infections to the skin rash?
5. What etiologic agents are suspect here?
6. How can you discount a skin allergy (contact dermatitis)?
7. What would the sanitation officer recommend to prevent a recurrence of this disease?
8. Is it necessary to treat the wrestling team members, and, if so, how?
9. What are the major characteristics of bacterial agents of dermatitis?
10. What virulence products are associated with the primary bacterial suspect of this case?

Student Questions

Case 3 Jack L. and Hide

Jack L. had recently accepted employment with the Western Tanning Company in Denver. This company purchased animal hides from slaughtering houses throughout the Rocky Mountain states. Jack worked as a receiving dock supervisor. He monitored shipments to the firm for the kind, quality, and number of hides received from their several suppliers. As a new employee, Jack was trying to impress his boss. He worked faithfully at his primary assignment and at times assisted clerks with their manual handling of the hides. Most of the hides were in a dry salt packing used to prevent spoilage, which tended to dry Jack's hands, since he didn't use gloves on those sporadic occasions when he helped the dock workers.

Two months after his employment, Jack noticed a small pustule had developed overnight on the back of his left hand. Within 2 days this had enlarged and was surrounded by a rim of extensive edema. Twenty-four hours later the center of this lesion collapsed. It had a wet, almost gelatinous appearance, and its center was dark, nearly black in color. Although this lesion was not painful, it was obviously not healing spontaneously, so Jack contacted his physician.

The physician examined a Gram stain taken from material collected from the center of the lesion. He expected to find a good population of large gram-positive bacilli but actually found only a few such bacteria. The absence of bacterial spores in the preparation was expected. A swab of the lesion was sent to the clinical laboratory for exact identification of the organism, but the physician had enough confidence in his ability to diagnose this disease that he began Jack on a regimen of penicillin.

Questions

1. What is (are) the name(s) of this skin lesion?
2. Is this disease common in the United States?
3. What species of animals are most often associated with this disease?
4. What are the typical routes of transmission of this disease?

5. How is the etiologic agent in this case distinguished from nonpathogenic species in the same genus?
6. What are the morphologic features of the pathogen in this case?
7. What is a Medusa-head colony?
8. Describe the toxin(s) that participate in this disease.
9. Is penicillin the best therapeutic?
10. Is there no vaccine against this disease?

Student Questions

Case 4 A Sore Spot

Tony had worked but 3 weeks at Gardendale Nursery when the sore first appeared on his left forearm. The work had not been that much of a challenge. Every day those first 2 weeks he had been mulching the rose bushes and smaller shrubs. The mulch came in 5-cubic foot plastic bags that were hard to move about. Shoveling the mulch in and around the rose bushes was especially aggravating because of all the tiny scratches he got on his arms.

The small sore on Tony's arm wasn't painful or even very red, and he thought it would probably go away in a day or two. But 3 days later Tony noticed a lump a little higher up his arm and a raised cord extending from the open sore to the lump. He told the nursery owner about it, and the owner remembered that a yard worker over at Floral Gardens Nursery had something like that a couple of years ago, but he couldn't recall exactly what it was. He told Tony to take the afternoon off and go see his doctor.

Tony's physician noted that his patient had no fever and was in obvious good health except for the small ulcer on his left arm. Microscopic examination did not visualize any microorganisms. Cultures from the lesion were positive for *Staphylococcus epidermidis* the next day, but no additional organisms were recovered after 48 hours' incubation of the specimen.

Questions

1. Is this typical of an infection by *Staphylococcus epidermidis*?
2. How does this lesion differ from that produced by *Francisella tularensis*?
3. What features of this disease indicate it is not of bacterial origin?
4. This disease seems like an occupational hazard. What other vocations are especially at risk?
5. If the true pathogen were seen in stains of the ulcerated lesion, how would it appear?
6. Would its appearance be the same in culture? In animal virulence tests?
7. Make a drawing of the pathogen, and label appropriately.
8. What culture technique(s) should be used to isolate the pathogen?
9. What are the therapeutic options?
10. What is the preferred therapy?

Student Questions

Case 5 The Chicken Farmer

Shortly after falling asleep, Barney G. awoke to a sound that he hated—the sound of panic in the chicken coop. Barney closed the coop up tightly every night and even checked around the foundation of the shed periodically to be certain no digging or burrowing animal could get in. Obviously something had happened.

Barney jumped from his bed, pulled on his trousers, stuffed his feet into his slippers, and headed out the back door of the farmhouse. On the back porch he picked up his flashlight and shotgun, which he loaded as he ran toward the chicken house. He threw open the door and saw the chickens jumping, thrashing about wildly as they tried to avoid an animal on the floor. At first Barney couldn't see what kind of an animal it was until he saw the white streak down the center of its broad black back. Barney brought the shotgun to his shoulder, but before he could pull the trigger he lost sight of the animal as it ran from the flashlight's beam. When Barney relocated the skunk, it was practically at his feet, too near for a safe shot, so he kicked at the animal. But the skunk was too fast for him—it bit him on the ankle, released its bite as Barney kicked at it with his other foot, and disappeared into the darkness.

It was all too clear what would happen tomorrow—a drive to town, a visit with Doc Swanson, and probably another one of those "serum shots" that made him swell up like a balloon after that tractor accident 4 years ago.

Questions

1. What kind of "serum shot" did think Barney receive after his tractor accident?
2. What was the nature of his allergic response at that time? Explain in detail.
3. Would Barney receive the same kind of "serum shot" after an animal bite?
4. What diseases are transmissible by bites of a skunk or other wild animal?
5. Name and describe the etiologic agent in each case.
6. What is the treatment for each of the diseases listed in response to question 4?
7. Will Doc Swanson actively immunize Barney against any diseases, and if so, which diseases?
8. What undomesticated animals are the primary source of human infections?
9. Are any zoonoses uniformly fatal?
10. Where does serology fit into the diagnosis of animal bite infections?

Student Questions

Case 6 The Naughty Neighbor

Mandy, a 4-year-old, watched hopefully next door as the truck unloaded. Three men steadily carried a tricycle, a wagon, a swing set, other toys, lamps, furniture, and other household goods into the house next door. All this was done under the direction of a woman who looked almost like Mandy's mother, but as yet no children could be seen to go with the swing set, wagon, or tricycle.

Mandy's wait wasn't long. Before the truck was emptied, a man arrived in a station wagon with two children near Mandy's age. As they stepped out of the car, Mandy went to greet them. One of the girls had a cat in her arms, and when Mandy went to pet the cat, the animal scratched Mandy's hand and bit her on the right index finger.

Of course, Mandy cried out, bringing both her mother and the neighbor lady to the scene. The apologies were profuse. The neighbor assured them that the cat had all her shots and there was no danger of rabies. Fortunately the bite was only on the index finger of Mandy's right hand, and only a few drops of blood were lost.

Five days later Mandy's finger, which at first seemed to be healing, was red, swollen, and throbbing. When the family pediatrician saw the finger and heard of the cat bite, he indicated that any of several bacteria could be the cause. He collected a little of the wound drainage on a swab for culture and prescribed a broad-spectrum antibiotic. He said it would be a day or two before he could be certain about the cause of the lesion but to call if Mandy showed any signs of a more serious illness.

Questions

1. Is this a typical progression of cat-scratch fever?
2. What agents did the pediatrician have in mind when he said several agents could be involved?
3. How are erysipelas, erysipeloid, and cat-scratch fever distinguished microbiologically?
4. What "shots" are given to cats and dogs?
5. Describe rabies vaccines.
6. What antibiotics are recommended in this case?
7. Are animals other than cats implicated in cat-scratch fever?
8. Mandy apparently had no significant generalized symptoms of disease. Explain.
9. Is there an explanation of why the bite became infected and not the scratches on Mandy's hand?
10. What prophylactic measures should Mandy's mother have used to prevent this situation?

Student Questions

Case 7 Fishing for an Answer

Lucia, the 19-year-old daughter of Emilia G., had worked with her mother in the family fish market only a few weeks after leaving her position as a cashier in a nearby supermarket. She enjoyed being a part of the family business despite the fact that it was a more demanding job than punching keys on a cash register. Also disturbing was the fact that her hands seemed always to be in water and had gradually taken on the classic dry, red look of dishwasher's hands. She applied lotion regularly and began to wear plastic gloves more faithfully to protect her hands.

Last Saturday the index finger on her left hand was "inoculated" by the dorsal fin of a bluefish she was cleaning. Over the weekend the area round the puncture remained red. On Monday no particular change could be noted, but by Friday the area had become larger, was painful and swollen, and had taken on a violet-red hue. It was apparent to her and to her mother that she had some type of an infection. She made an appointment later that day at her health management organization clinic.

Questions

1. How does this situation differ from the previous case in terms of probable etiology?
2. Is this lesion typical of any particular pathogen?
3. Does the agent responsible for this human disease actually cause disease in fish?
4. What culture characteristics are typical of the pathogen in this case?
5. How do the terms *erysipelas* and *erysipeloid* relate to this case?
6. What therapy is recommended here?
7. What prophylactic measures would have minimized the chance for this condition to develop?
8. Does a protective immunity develop against this disease after the primary infection so that Lucia won't contract this disease again?

Student Questions

Case 8 What a Blast

Jamal B., a 21-year-old, black construction worker had worked faithfully at his job despite the heat and dust of that North Carolina summer. Early in June he had a light summer cold but had never missed a day of work. Since that time he still had occasional chest pains and was often tired. He had also lost about 4 pounds. He attributed this to the fact that he was doing hard manual labor, including a lot of overtime. He had also slept through a few breakfasts and on those days had little time to fix a decent lunch pail. All of this probably accounted for his weight loss.

Now, just after the Fourth of July celebration, he noted several small swollen nodules on his forehead. At first he thought these were just pimples, but they steadily increased in size over the next week. At that time, he noticed a lump just under the skin of his right forearm, and within another week this ulcerated and began to drain.

His physician found Jamal to be a well-muscled young man, still in his normal weight range, though stating that he had recently lost 4 or 5 pounds. His lung x-ray indicated an infiltration of the right upper lobe, which was compatible with decreased breath sounds from the same area. Hematologic studies revealed a normal white cell count and differential. Jamal's hematocrit was 38%, and his hemoglobin 10.7 g/dl.

Material taken from the draining ulcer was sent to the laboratory with a request for routine tests plus cultures for fungi.

Questions

1. What is the presumptive diagnosis? A systemic infection expressed in the skin suggests what pathogens?
2. Could this be an atypical mycobacterial infection?
3. Describe the microbiologic diagnosis of atypical mycobacterial infections.
4. What fungal infections are possible here?
5. What therapy is recommended if this is a fungal disease?
6. What procedures should be used to recover fungi from a draining abscess?
7. What is the route of entry of most fungal diseases?
8. What immunologic studies might prove useful in this case?
9. Describe the fungi that cause systemic infections.
10. Describe the use of antibiotics in media used to culture fungi.

Student Questions

Case 9 Cellulitis

As Sandy gradually awoke from an afternoon nap while sunbathing on her deck, she felt something move on the back of her left hand. As she brushed at her hand, she felt a sharp sting and then saw the partially crushed bee.

Sandy entered the house, put a few ice cubes in a washcloth, and placed them on the area of the sting, which was already red and slightly swollen. That evening the inflammation on the back of her hand had increased slightly and was still very evident when Sandy went to work the next morning. By 11 AM, Sandy noted that her hand was swollen so badly that she couldn't close her fist easily. Her fingers were also swelling, and a red streak was forming on the underside of her left forearm.

Sandy went to the employee's clinic, where she was told she had an infection. She was given a prescription for erythromycin and told to go home, to rest, and to keep her hand elevated. She was asked to return the next morning for an evaluation.

On Tuesday morning, her condition was perhaps slightly better, certainly not any worse, and the doctors repeated their earlier instructions. That evening she noted that her hand and fingers were not as swollen and the redness on her forearm had diminished.

Questions

1. This disease erupted quickly after the bee sting. Do bees carry human pathogens?
2. What aspects of the reaction to bee stings favor the later developments of the condition seen in this case?
3. Is this an infection caused by an endogenous organism? Explain your position.
4. What toxic properties of bacteria permit this type of an illness to develop?
5. What will Sandy's immune status be to reinfection after recovery?
6. Will any permanent after-effect result from this illness?
7. What data argue against this being the early stages of gas gangrene?
8. Describe the bacterial flora of healthy skin.
9. Why was no specimen or serum collected to help determine the exact diagnosis?

Student Questions

Review Questions

1. Dimorphic fungi are the etiologic agents of all the following **except**
   A. Histoplasmosis
   B. Dermatophytosis
   C. Sporotrichosis
   D. Coccidioidomycosis
   E. Blastomycosis

2. Which of the following is the most communicable person to person?
   A. Gas gangrene
   B. Sporotrichosis
   C. Tinea capitis
   D. Herpetic whitlow
   E. Erysipeloid

3. The causative agent of human erysipelas is
   A. Also the cause of erysipeloid
   B. *Erysipelothrix rhusiopathiae*
   C. *Streptococcus pyogenes*
   D. Also the cause of erythrasma
   E. The only known species in its genus

4. The disease acne is caused by
   A. *Propionibacterium*
   B. *Staphylococcus*
   C. The same bacteria that cause swimmer's itch
   D. *Epidermophyton floccosum*
   E. None of the above

5. Deep wound infections are usually responsible for
   A. Gas gangrene
   B. Short incubation time rabies
   C. Tetanus
   D. Osteomyelitis
   E. All of the above

6. Which of the following is least likely to be caused by staphylococci?
   A. Cellulitis
   B. Scalded skin syndrome
   C. Postpartum endometriosis
   D. Furuncles
   E. Impetigo

7. Which of the following viruses is least associated with a skin eruption?

A. Herpes simplex
B. Mumps
C. Variola
D. Molluscum contagiosum
E. Varicella

8. A puncture wound from a thorny plant is often associated with

A. Tularemia
B. Tetanus
C. Erysipelas
D. Sporotrichosis
E. Herpes zoster

9. Most dermatophytic fungal diseases

A. Are due to dimorphic agents
B. Are in the genus *Epidermophyton*
C. Involve both nails and hair
D. Are treatable with amphotericin B
E. None of the above

10. Tetanus

A. Is caused by several antigenic forms of tetanospasmin
B. Like botulism and gas gangrene is caused by a soil inhabitant
C. Immunization provides protection via the content of antitoxin in the vaccine
D. Is the result of an intoxication in the absence of an infection
E. Umbilicus is not caused by *Clostridium tetani*

7 Diseases of the Central Nervous System

Infectious diseases of the central nervous system (CNS) are often initially contracted as airborne diseases. Following or accompanying an upper respiratory tract infection, a bacteremia develops. Transgression of the blood-brain barrier then leads to meningitis, encephalitis, or a brain abscess. Many viruses enter the CNS through this pathway and cause encephalitis. Typical of the primary bacterial agents of meningitis are *Haemophilus influenzae*, *Neisseria meningitidis*, and *Streptococcus pneumoniae*. Gram-negative anaerobes are prominent among bacteria causing brain abscesses.

A neuronal avenue to the CNS is used by the rabies virus, tetanus toxin, and possibly botulinum toxin, although the blood route is more likely for the last.

The diagnostic approach for diseases of the CNS begins with the realization that representatives of all groups of microbes—bacteria, fungi, viruses, rickettsiae, spirochetes, amoebae, even nematodes and cestodes—may be involved (Table 7-1). Secondly, a consideration of the selective ability of certain microbes to affect special age groups or other special populations is important. For example, group B streptococci

Table 7-1. Major etiologic agents of central nervous system diseases

Disease	Agent
Acute meningitis	*Escherichia coli*
	Haemophilus influenzae, type b
	Group B streptococci
	Neisseria meningitidis
	Streptococcus pneumoniae
	Enteroviruses
Encephalitis	Herpes simplex virus
	Arbovirus
	Enterovirus
Brain abscess	*Staphylococcus aureus*
	Bacteroides species
Chronic nervous system disease	HIV-1
	Treponema pallidum
	Cryptococcus neoformans

and *Escherichia coli* are far more frequent in very young infants than in other age groups. *Haemophilus*, *Neisseria,* and *S. pneumoniae* affect older children and young adults. Immunocompromised patients represent a special group that are susceptible to feeble pathogens such as the yeast *Cryptococcus neoformans.*

The major diagnostic aid is probably the analysis of cerebrospinal fluid (CSF). This fluid is normally clear, contains less than 10 cells/μl, most of which will be lymphocytes, and contains glucose at 50 to 80 mg/dl (Table 7-2). Deviations from these figures include decreased levels of glucose as an index of bacterial and fungal infections, and normal levels as more compatible with a viral etiology. Increased numbers of lymphocytes suggest viral or fungal infections or tuberculous meningitis. Bacterial infections draw neutrophils into the CSF at cell counts up to 10,000/μl. In most cases of meningitis, the CSF will be hazy as a result of these cellular infiltrates.

Brain abscesses present a slightly different profile of these values. Usually the blood glucose level is normal in a mixed population of cells that may include plasma cells. The CSF fluid may be either clear or turbid. Neurosyphilis deviates from these generalities notably by having a normal glucose level, having little or no increase in lymphocytes, and presenting as a clear fluid.

The microorganisms that cause these diseases may be visualized in direct stains of the CSF, but stains of the sediment of centrifuged CSF are more productive. These should include acid-fast as well as Gram stains. Special techniques (India ink wet mount preparations, serologic tests for antigens in the CSF) are useful in certain circumstances.

Because of the seriousness of acute CNS disease, an early correct diagnosis and application of the appropriate chemotherapy are necessary to prevent the development of undesirable neuropathologic sequelae.

Key Words and Phrases

This checklist of key words, phrases, and abbreviations has been subdivided in a different format than any used earlier. Remember to make your own additions as you encounter new terms.

MICROBE DATA

Alpha hemolysis
Acid-fast
Beta hemolysis
Bile solubility test
Capsular antigen vaccine
Chocolate agar
Coliform
Cord factor
Group B streptococci
India ink wet mount
Lactose fermenter
Lancefield grouping
Löwenstein–Jensen medium
Optochin
Oxidase test
Satellite phenomenon
Thayer–Martin medium

Tuberculin
Wassermann test
Ziehl–Neelsen stain

DISEASE

Aedes species
Aseptic meningitis
Culex tarsalis
Dermacentor species
Herpetic whitlow
Postinfectious encephalitis
Postvaccinal encephalitis
Purulent meningitis
Sentinel bird
Tick fever
Waterhouse–Friderichsen syndrome

Table 7-2. Values of cerebrospinal fluid in various infectious conditions

Condition	Appearance	Cellularity	Glucose level
Normal	Clear	0–5/µl, lymphocytes	50–80 mg/dl
Bacterial meningitis	Cloudy	1,000–10,000 neutrophils	Decreased
Fungal meningitis	Hazy or clear	Increased, lymphocytes	Decreased
Viral meningitis	Clear or hazy	Increased, lymphocytes	Normal
Abscess	Cloudy	Increased, mixed population	Normal
Neurosyphilis	Clear	Slight increase in lymphocytes	Normal

Abbreviations

BCG
CSF-VDRL
EEE
FTA-ABS
K antigen
OT
PPD
RPR
SLE
TPI
VCN medium
VDRL
V factor
WEE
X factor

Information Sources

Booss, J., and Esiri, M.: Viral encephalitis: pathology, diagnosis, and management, Blackwell Scientific, 1986, Oxford.

Evans, A.S., editor: Viral infections of humans: epidemiology and control, edition 3, Plenum Press, Inc., 1991, New York.

Evans, A.S., and Brachman, P.S., editors: Bacterial infections of humans: epidemiology and control, edition 2, Plenum Press, Inc., 1991, New York.

Finegold, S.M., and George, W.L., editors: Anaerobic infections in humans, Academic Press, Inc., 1989, San Diego.

Grange, J.M.: Mycobacteria and human disease, Edward Arnold, 1988, London.

Monath, T.P., editor: The arboviruses: epidemiology and ecology, vol. 1–5, CRC Press, 1989, Boca Raton.

Poolman, J.T.: Gonococci and meningococci, Kluwer Academic Publishers, 1988, Dordrecht.

Roizman, B., editor: Herpesviruses, vol. I and II, Plenum Publishing Co., 1982, New York.

Sande, M.A., Smith, A.L., and Root, R.K., editors: Bacterial meningitis, Churchill Livingstone, 1985, New York.

Scheld, W.M., Whitely, R.J., and Durack, D.T., editors: Infections of the central nervous system, Raven Press, Inc., 1991, New York.

Schlesinger, S., and Schlesinger, M.J., editors: The Togaviridae and Flaviviridae, Plenum Publishing Co., 1986, New York.

Sell, S.H., and Wright, P.F.: *Haemophilus influenzae*: epidemiology, immunology, and prevention of disease, Elsevier Biomedical, 1982, New York.

Simpson, L.L., editor: Botulinum neurotoxin and tetanus toxin, Academic Press, Inc., 1989, San Diego.

Specter, S., Bendinelli, M., and Friedman, H., editors: Neuropathogenic viruses and immunity, Plenum Publishing Co., 1992, New York.

Case 1 Mallory's Malady

Mallory, a 5-year-old girl, was brought by police ambulance to an emergency room of a suburban community hospital on the evening of December 4. She was acutely ill, irritable, and incoherent on admission. According to her parents, she had been seen by her pediatrician for the croup 4 days earlier and was now receiving ampicillin orally. The child had complained of a headache that morning, had vomited her breakfast soon after eating, and had a temperature of 101°F at that time. By early afternoon, she had become increasingly irritable and complained that her head hurt and that it hurt her neck when she turned her head. By the dinner hour, Mallory's temperature had risen to 104°F, she became incoherent and began to exhibit severe flexion spasms of the head and neck, and she was transferred immediately to the emergency room.

Physical examination of the child in the emergency room revealed a cherry-red epiglottis, temperature of 104°F, and a blood pressure of 150/60 mm Hg. The lungs appeared clear, and the heart seemed normal with no evidence of murmurs. Her neck was stiff, and even a small degree of dorsiflexion was impossible.

Immediate lumbar puncture was performed with the patient securely restrained. The CSF was moderately cloudy and contained 15,000 leukocytes/mm^3, of which 94% were segmented neutrophils. The CSF glucose was decreased (25 mg/dl) with simultaneous blood glucose at 194 mg/dl, and the CSF protein level was elevated. A Gram stain of the centrifuged CSF sediment failed to reveal bacteria.

Questions

1. What is the relationship of croup to meningitis?
2. Describe the etiology of croup.
3. Do the data for the CSF suggest a bacterial or viral etiology?

4. No bacteria were seen in Gram stains of CSF sediment. Explain.
5. What culture procedures should be used in an effort to recover bacteria?
6. What bacteria and viruses are most common in meningitis of preschool-age children?
7. What is the genetic basis of ampicillin resistance in bacteria?
8. What antibiotics are recommended for the treatment of early childhood, ampicillin-resistant meningitis?
9. Describe the Waterhouse-Friderichsen syndrome in detail.
10. How would you treat viral meningitis?

Student Questions

Case 2 An Early Demise

A 17-day-old black female infant was brought to the hospital by her mother. Both the mother and child had appeared well at discharge 13 days earlier. The mother said that since that time her baby had not nursed well but did not appear unusually fussy or ill. However, the baby cried almost all last night and felt feverish to the mother, who had no thermometer to determine the extent of the fever. This morning she borrowed a thermometer from a neighbor and found that the child had a rectal temperature of 102.6°F. She planned to bring her baby to the hospital but tried to nurse her first. The baby took a little milk but soon vomited.

On examination in the emergency room, the baby was dehydrated and semidelirious. The vital signs were as follows:

Temperature (rectal)	103°F
Pulse	110
Respirations	13
Blood pressure	110/60 mm Hg

The lungs were clear, as were the ears, nose, and throat. Nuchal rigidity was obvious, so a spinal tap was ordered. The CSF findings were as follows:

Color	Slightly white and cloudy
Cells	1800 neutrophils
	20 lymphocytes
Glucose	20 mg/dl

Small gram-negative cells were found in some of the neutrophils collected from the CSF sediment. The attending intern could not definitely determine if the bacteria were cocci or short bacilli. Ampicillin and amikacin were begun immediately by IV.

Within 2 hours the child lapsed into unconsciousness, lost blood pressure, decreased respiration, and was intubated. One hour later the child expired.

Questions

1. Is the child's illness acquired from the mother, the hospital staff, the home environment, or where?
2. Is this most apt to be a bacterial infection by *Haemophilus*, *Neisseria*, or *Escherichia*? Explain. Could the Gram stain be in error?
3. Describe the bacterial spectrum of amikacin, and list related antibiotics.
4. What is the bacterial spectrum of ampicillin?
5. Did the Waterhouse-Friderichsen syndrome kill this child?
6. Would the satellite phenomenon help to recover these bacteria in culture? Explain this phenomenon.
7. Would you recommend prophylactic therapy for the mother and other contacts?
8. Do the CSF data pretty well eliminate tuberculous meningitis?

Student Questions

Case 3 Another Sick Baby

Dana had reached her 8-month birthday, but it was no party for her or her mother. For the last several days Dana had a runny nose and had been unusually fussy. This morning about 3 AM, she woke her mother with a siege of uncontrollable crying. Her rectal temperature was 101°F, so her mother gave her a cool bath. After the bath, the child fell asleep for only 20 or 30 minutes and began to cry again. As her mother tried to comfort her, Dana vomited. Her rectal temperature was now 102.8°F, so Dana's mother rushed her daughter to the hospital emergency room.

Data from the physical examination indicated that the child had an inflamed throat, bilateral swollen eardrums, and clear chest sound and that she cried whenever her neck was bent or turned.

A spinal tap was performed, and CSF and blood were sent for culture. The CSF was slightly cloudy, but only red cells and white cells were seen in Gram stains of the centrifuged pellet. The white blood cell count was elevated to 17,000/mm^3 and dominated by neutrophils. The CSF was sent to the laboratory for culture.

The physician prescribed combination drug therapy by the intravenous route for fear of ampicillin resistance in the etiologic agent.

Questions

1. What antibiotic combination should the physician in this case consider?
2. Bacteria were not seen in the CSF. Is this a viral disease? What data argue against that possibility?
3. What culture tests identify *Escherichia coli*? Group B streptococci?
4. What culture tests identify *Neisseria meningitidis*?
5. What culture tests identify *Haemophilus influenzae*?
6. How would you treat *E. coli* meningitis? Group B streptococcal meningitis?
7. What are the X and V factors?
8. How is chocolate agar prepared?
9. How does 5% carbon dioxide stimulate bacterial growth?
10. Does *Streptococcus pneumoniae* cause meningitis?
11. How—from what source—did Dana contract this infection?

Student Questions

Case 4 And Sick to Boot

Recruit Olson, an 18-year-old farm boy, had enlisted in the Navy as soon as the conflict had broken out. His first 2 weeks in boot camp had been rougher than he expected. Running the obstacle course in soft sand, swimming twice the pool length in full gear, rowing the old-fashioned whale boat with only three others at the oars, and other physical fitness challenges had built him up and torn him down at the same time. He was physically fit but constantly tired.

His bout with "cat fever," the trainees' term for catarrhal fever, was starting to get the best of him. A few days ago it was just a mild sore throat and runny nose, but now he had a nice, pounding frontal headache. The aching shoulders and stiff neck he had when he woke up didn't seem so bad now, but he decided to check into the sick bay anyway.

Lieutenant Lewis made a routine physical examination and found that Recruit Olson had painful draining sinuses with a purulent discharge, an inflamed pharynx, and slight nuchal rigidity, but lungs, abdomen, and extremities were normal. Vital signs were as follows:

Temperature	99.9°F
Pulse	71
Blood pressure	129/82 mm Hg
Respirations	20

Lieutenant Lewis collected a nasopharyngeal swab, retained Recruit Olson in the sick bay for further observation, and called the Medical Quartermaster's office to inquire about the vaccine inventory.

Questions

1. What is the expected normal flora recovered via nasopharyngeal swabs?
2. Are there any specific pathogens associated with cat fever?
3. What is Thayer-Martin VCN medium?
4. How is chocolate agar prepared, and what is its advantage over ordinary blood agar?
5. Explain the basis and specificity of the oxidase test.
6. What vaccine stock was of interest to Lieutenant Lewis?
7. What treatment should Recruit Olson receive?
8. Discuss prophylactic chemotherapy in terms of this case.
9. What vaccines would you recommend for military recruits?
10. What is the relative status of *Streptococcus pneumoniae* and *Neisseria meningitis* in this case?

Student Questions

Case 5 No Car Meningitis

When you hit an oil patch on the asphalt at 125 miles per hour in the first turn, the inevitable will happen. Larry E., a 38-year-old race car driver, regained consciousness 2 days later. Through his drug-shrouded mind he eventually learned what happened. It was miraculous that he had only seven broken bones rather evenly distributed from his ankle to the cranium. In some ways the concussion was the worst part of it because the Racing Commission would put him through some rigid tests before he could go out on the track again.

Larry's delay in returning to the pits was much longer than he expected. Five weeks after his crash, while recuperating at home, he began to develop a headache and stiff neck. Within 2 days he developed a fever of 101°F, and on the next day he vomited and acted confused. He was taken to the local hospital where the emergency room doctors noted these symptoms and ordered a spinal tap. The CSF contained 872 WBCs/mm^3, of which 82% were polymorphonuclear neutrophil leukocytes. Since a bacterial meningitis was suspected, CSF was sent to the laboratory for culture, and the patient was begun on ampicillin.

After 8 days, Larry's condition had not improved significantly, so therapy was changed to chloramphenicol. There was still no improvement noted by day 18 of hospitalization. On day 20, amphotericin B therapy replaced chloramphenicol, since Larry was now in a severely weakened condition and the antibacterial antibiotics were ineffective.

On day 30, the laboratory reported that CSF cultures were positive for gram-positive, weakly acid-fast, filamentous, branching bacilli. On this basis, the therapy was again changed, to trimethoprim-sulfamethoxazole and minocycline. This therapy was continued for 6 months, and only then would the Racing Commission re-instate Larry's license.

Questions

1. What acid-fast organisms cause meningitis?
2. Describe the Ziehl–Neelsen stain.
3. What are the major components of Löwenstein-Jensen medium?
4. Does the therapy chosen show good activity against all acid-fast organisms?
5. How do you explain the failure of the physician to perform skin tests?
6. Define photochromogen, scotochromogen, and nonchromogen.
7. Why was amphotericin B chosen early in the course of this disease?
8. How is a head injury associated with meningitis? Where does the pathogen come from?
9. What other diseases are caused by the pathogens under consideration in this case?
10. Do animal parasites ever cause meningitis? Explain.

Student Questions

Case 6 Too Old to Count

Ben F., a 50-year-old bachelor, failed to report for work in the diagnostic bacteriology laboratory on Monday morning. When no one answered the phone at Ben's apartment, Susan, the laboratory supervisor, voiced concern about Ben's health. For the last 2 weeks, Ben had been working on a research project for the State Health Laboratory. A collection of *Streptococcus pyogenes*, *Streptococcus pneumoniae*, and *Staphylococcus aureus* cultures from recent cases of meningitis in nursing homes had been sent to the laboratory for analysis. Ben had been evaluating these cultures for several virulence properties. Unfortunately, only 2 days after he began work on the project, Ben developed a slight cold.

About 10 o'clock, when repeated calls to Ben's apartment had gone unanswered, Sue received a CSF specimen from the emergency room. She was shocked when she saw Ben's name on the specimen. A Gram stain of the CSF sediment revealed gram-positive cocci.

Questions

1. Laboratory-acquired infections with pathogenic cocci are relatively rare. Are there any factors that would lead you to believe this is such an infection?
2. Does the incubation time of meningitis due to gram-positive bacteria agree with your answer to question 1?
3. What is the correlation of age group with the etiology of bacterial meningitis?
4. What are the major virulence properties of *S. pyogenes*?
5. Discuss the role of antistreptolysin assays in streptococcal disease.
6. What are the major virulence properties of *S. aureus*?
7. What are the major virulence properties of *S. pneumoniae*?
8. Why are vaccines effective against *S. pneumoniae*, but not against *S. pyogenes*?
9. How do you identify pathogenic staphylococci in the laboratory?
10. How do you distinguish *S. pneumoniae* from other alpha-hemolytic streptococci?

Student Questions

Case 7 Tina's Trouble

Tina, a 10-month-old girl, had become ill over the past 4 or 5 days. She had diarrhea for the first 2 days, but this had subsided more recently. Her rectal temperature had been elevated but not enough to cause much concern. She never seemed to finish her bottle, was irritable, and didn't sleep well. Now that she was developing a skin rash, Tina's mother decided her baby needed a medical examination.

Dr. Davis was perplexed by his findings. He had detected a possible bulging fontanelle but no other neurologic abnormalities. The rash was not pathognomonic of any viral infection of childhood. Vital signs—body temperature and respirations—were only mildly elevated. Dr. Davis requested peripheral blood studies and, more on a hunch than actual evidence, ordered a spinal fluid tap.

The hematology laboratory reported 11,200 WBCs/mm^3, of which 56% were neutrophils and 36% were lymphocytes. The CSF had 32% neutrophils and 31% monocytes of the 600 WBCs/mm^3. The glucose value was normal, and the protein was slightly elevated. Bacterial cultures of blood and CSF remained negative. Dr. Davis made the unusual request for a second spinal tap to send to the State Health Laboratory for possible virus identification.

Questions

1. Do any of the blood or CSF values suggest a CNS viral disease?
2. What are the common agents of viral meningitis and encephalitis?
3. Which of these are most commonly seen in young children?
4. What is the relative role of cell culture isolation of viruses versus serologic diagnosis of viral meningitis?
5. What is the role of newborn mice in the diagnosis of viral meningitis?
6. Is a fungal meningitis outside the realm of possibilities in this case?
7. If this were a case of tuberculous meningitis, what would be your position on skin tests and therapy for Tina and her family members?
8. What is your definition of aseptic meningitis?
9. Is there any suitable therapy for viral meningoencephalitis?
10. What are the sequelae of viral meningoencephalitis?

Student Questions

Case 8 An Iatrogenic Illness

Gregory's life had been filled with medical experiences. As a young boy, he had pneumonia twice in the pre-antibiotic era. Fortunately the sulfa drugs had just become available and had probably saved his life. The same could be claimed for his case of scarlet fever, although he might have recovered from all of these infections with good luck.

He escaped the Korean conflict with a slight shrapnel wound and the usual respiratory infections of wintertime warfare in a cold climate.

Greg's health record in the 1960s and 70s wasn't unusual—a couple of incidents of traveler's diarrhea in Mexico, some intestinal polyps that were removed, as well as nasal polyps that were removed on two occasions. The nasal polyps didn't recur after he quit smoking.

Now Greg was diagnosed as having Hodgkin's disease and was started on cytotoxic drug therapy. One month after treatment was initiated, he began to have some mild headaches and occasional dizziness. These became more serious over the next 2 weeks, and he complained to his doctor at his regular checkup.

At this time, the physician noted that Greg had an unsteady gait and was slow to respond to questions about the increasing severity of his headaches. His doctor thought Greg might have meningitis, even though he had no fever and no stiff neck. A lumbar tap yielded CSF that was low in glucose (34 mg/dl) and elevated in protein (600 mg/dl). Mononuclear cells were elevated. The Gram stain revealed no bacteria, but numerous aberrant staining cells resembling lymphocytes were seen.

Further laboratory studies to confirm a diagnosis of meningitis were ordered.

Questions

1. Explain how cytotoxic drug therapy can lead to meningitis.
2. Is this most likely a viral, bacterial, or fungal disease? Why?
3. Which viral agents are associated with meningitis?
4. How is viral meningitis treated?
5. What fungi are associated with meningitis?
6. How is fungal meningitis treated?
7. Define chronic and acute meningitis.
8. Do any of Greg's earlier bacterial illnesses relate to either Hodgkin's disease or meningitis?
9. How are cultures for fungi conducted in the laboratory?
10. Compare yeasts, dimorphic fungi, and molds from the viewpoint of structure and growth.

Student Questions

Review Questions

1. Which of the following statements regarding infection caused by the meningococcus is false?
   A. It is often asymptomatic or only results in a mild nasopharyngitis.
   B. It can produce a meningococcemia with a petechial rash.
   C. It may spread in epidemic fashion in overcrowded conditions.
   D. *Neisseria meningitidis* is presumptively diagnosed by finding intracellular gram-negative diplococci in polymorphonuclear neutrophil leukocytes in the spinal fluid.
   E. No vaccine is available for prevention of meningococcal infection.

2. Cryptococcal meningitis is caused by
   A. A dimorphic fungus
   B. A monomorphic fungus
   C. A multiple budding yeast
   D. A parasite in the genus *Coccidia*
   E. None of the above

3. The major causative agent of meningitis in infants less than 1 month old is
   A. *Neisseria meningitidis*
   B. *Haemophilus influenzae*, type b
   C. *Streptococcus pneumoniae*
   D. *Escherichia coli*
   E. *Staphylococcus aureus*

4. An encapsulated yeast seen in India ink preparations of CSF is most probably
   A. *Mycobacterium tuberculosis*
   B. *Cryptococcus neoformans*
   C. *Coccidioides immitis*
   D. *Candida albicans*
   E. *Histoplasma capsulatum*

5. The vaccine against *Neisseria meningitidis* infections
   A. Is composed of RPR
   B. Is protective only against serotype B organisms
   C. Is ineffective in children less than 18 months of age
   D. Is also protective against *Neisseria gonorrhoeae*
   E. Consists of whole killed cells of *N. meningitidis*

6. *Bacteroides* species
   A. Seldom cause meningitis but are a common cause of brain abscesses
   B. Are gram-negative anaerobic bacteria
   C. Are usually deficient in superoxide dismutase and catalase or peroxidase
   D. Are a common cause of aspiration pneumonia
   E. All of the above

7. Tuberculous meningitis is

A. Typically a subacute or chronic disease in contrast to most other bacterial meningitides
B. Best treated with a combination of antibacterial agents
C. Prone to cause a mononuclear lymphocytic infiltration of the CSF
D. Often diagnosed by culturing sputum, urine, or gastric aspirates as well as CSF
E. All of the above

8. Which of the following can cause aseptic meningitis?

A. *Leptospira interrogans*
B. Echoviruses
C. Poliomyelitis virus
D. Mumps vaccine
E. All of the above

9. The most common cause of aseptic meningitis is

A. Mumps virus
B. Echoviruses
C. Herpes virus
D. Influenza virus
E. *Leptospira interrogans*

10. Which of the following causes most of the cases of meningitis in adults?

A. *Streptococcus pneumoniae*
B. *Neisseria meningitidis*
C. *Streptococcus pyogenes*
D. *Staphylococcus aureus*
E. *Treponema pallidum*

8 Zoonoses

The zoonoses are infectious diseases of humans acquired from lower animals. The lower animal is usually a mammal but may be a bird. If a snail or arthropod is an intermediary in the life cycle of an infectious agent, such as a worm, that infects only humans, the disease is not typically considered a zoonosis. Both domesticated and wild animals are sources of zoonotic diseases. Obviously diseases contracted from wild animals are the more difficult to control, but because of restricted human contact with these animals, the diseases they transmit seldom reach epidemic proportions. Immunization, slaughter, food inspection, and pasteurization are used to control zoonoses of domestic animals.

There are five major avenues for transmission of zoonoses to humans: direct contact, inhalation, ingestion of contaminated foods, milk or milk products, animal bites, and insect vectors. In some instances after a human infection has developed, human-to-human transmission may occur. Plague is an example of animal-to-human-to-human transmission. An individual infectious agent may be transmitted by more than one route. For example, tularemia may be acquired by direct contact with an infected animal, ingestion of improperly prepared food, or the bite of an infected insect vector. Special problems are encountered in the control of the vector-borne zoonoses, since this requires control of both the wild animal source and the vector. Vector-borne zoonoses are considered in Chapter 9.

Since a close association with lower animals or animal products is the source of zoonotic diseases, a carefully taken patient history is useful in their diagnosis. Zoonoses are an occupational hazard for veterinarians, farmers, slaughterhouse workers, and kennel managers. Persons dwelling in rural areas are more apt to encounter diseased animals than those from urban centers. Certain ethnic groups may be at a higher risk if they have special dietary practices—eating raw or undercooked foods, or home preparation and consumption of ethnic foods. A recognition of these factors aids in the identification of the disease source and may assist in the prevention of further cases. Unfortunately, the breadth of etiologic agents involved in the zoonoses requires the practitioner to consider bacteria, viruses, and all other classes of microbes to establish the diagnosis.

The listing in Table 8-1 includes the zoonoses of North America. Fortunately, some of these—glanders, rabies, tapeworm, and several others—are quite rare.

Table 8-1. Zoonotic diseases of North America transmitted by other than arthropods

Disease	Animal source(s)	Means of transmission	Etiologic agent
Anthrax	Sheep, goats, cattle, most other domestic animals	Inhalation, direct contact, less often by ingestion	*Bacillus anthracis* spores
Brucellosis	Sheep, goats, swine, cattle, most other domestic animals	Raw milk, direct contact	*Brucella melitensis* *Brucella abortus* *Brucella suis*
Cat-scratch fever	Cats or dogs	Animal scratch	Rochalimaea-like organism
Cryptosporidiosis	Calves	Direct contact	*Cryptosporidium parvum*
Cutaneous larva migrans	Dogs, cats	Direct contact	*Ancylostoma braziliense* and other species
Echinococcosis	Sheep to dog and other canines	Canine feces	*Echinococcus granulosus* *Echinococcus multilocularis*
Erysipeloid	Fish, cattle	Puncture wound	*Erysipelothrix rhusiopathiae*
Dermatophytosis	Dogs, cats, horses, cattle	Direct contact	*Microsporum* or *Trichophyton* species
Glanders	Horses	Direct contact	*Pseudomonas mallei*
Leptospirosis	Dogs, rats, mice, cattle, swine, wild animals	Contact with urine-contaminated water	*Leptospira interrogans*
Listeriosis	Cattle, sheep, horses, birds, rodents	Ingestion, direct contact	*Listeria monocytogenes*
Lymphocytic choriomeningitis	Mice, rats, dogs	Inhalation	Arbovirus
Pasteurellosis	Rats, mice, cattle, sheep, swine	Animal bite	*Pasteurella multocida*
Psittacosis	Birds	Fecal aerosol	*Chlamydia psittaci*
Q fever	Sheep, goats, cattle	Inhalation	*Coxiella burnetii*
Rabies	Dogs, bats, skunks, cats	Animal bite	Rhabdovirus (rabies virus)
Salmonellosis	Mice, rats, chickens, turtles, most domestic animals	Ingestion, direct contact	*Salmonella enteritidis* *Salmonella typhimurium*, and other species
Tapeworm infection	Cattle and swine	Undercooked meat	*Taenia saginata* (beef) *Taenia solium* (pork)
Toxoplasmosis	Cats	Ingestion	*Toxoplasma gondii*
Tuberculosis	Cattle	Contaminated milk, direct contact	*Mycobacterium bovis*
Tularemia	Wild rabbits	Direct contact	*Francisella tularensis*
Trichinosis	Swine	Ingestion	*Trichinella spiralis*
Visceral larva migrans	Dogs, cats	Ingestion	*Toxocara canis* and other species

Key Words and Phrases

The listing in Table 8-1 includes animal parasites, both single and multicellular, several bacteria, fungi, and viruses. An understanding of a large vocabulary is necessary to discuss these agents intelligently. Fortunately, many of these terms have been encountered earlier in this book. Terms that apply primarily to arthropod-borne zoonoses are covered in Chapter 9.

BACTERIA AND VIRUSES

Arbovirus
Cold enrichment cultures
Dye inhibition test
Elementary body
Erysipeloid
Febrile agglutinins
H antigen
MacConkey agar
Malignant pustule
Negri body
O antigen
Pasteurization
Q fever
Rabbit fever
Reticulate body
Undulant fever
Weil's disease
Woolsorters' disease

FUNGI

Arthroconidia
Dermatophyte
Ectothrix infection
Endothrix infection
Macroconidia
Microconidia
Ringworm
Septate hypha
Tinea corporis, tinea pedis, tinea barbae, tinea capitis, tinea cruris, etc.

ANIMAL PARASITES

Armed tapeworm
Cyst
Cysticercus
Cysticercoid
Dye inhibition test
Encapsulated cyst
Gametocyte
Hydatid cyst
Merozoite
Oocyst
Sabin-Feldman dye test
Scolex
Sporozoite
Tachyzoite
Trophozoite
Zygote

Abbreviations

EF
HE agar
LCM
LF
LPS
PA
SS agar
TORCH
TSI
TWAR
XLD agar

Information Sources

Andrewes, C.H.: Viral and bacterial diagnoses, Bailliere Tindall, 1977, London.

Lincoln, R.E., and Fish, D.G.: Anthrax toxin, in Microbial toxins, vol. 3, by Montie, T.C., Kadis, S., and Ajl, S.J., editors, Academic Press, Inc., 1970, New York.

Madkour, M.M., editor: Brucellosis, Butterworth, 1989, London.

Miller, A.J., Smith, J.L., and Somkuti, G.A., editors: Foodborne listeriosis, Elsevier, 1990, New York.

Reeve, P., editor: Chlamydial infections, Springer-Verlag, 1987, New York.

Schachter, J., and Dawson, C.R.: Human chlamydial infections, PSG Publishing Company, 1978, Littleton, Mass.

Schnurrenberger, P.R.: An outline of the zoonoses, Iowa State University Press, 1981, Ames.

Seeliger, H.P.R.: Listeriosis, edition 2, Hafner, 1961, New York.

Weber, D.J., and Weinberg, A.N., editors: Animal-associated human infections, Infect. Dis. Clin. North Am. **5**(1):1, 1991.

Young, E.J., and Corbel, M.J.: Brucellosis: clinical and laboratory aspects, CRC Press, 1989, Boca Raton.

Case 1 Cheese/Rabbit

Bobby Jack, a 17-year-old Arkansas farm boy, was glad to see the light snow outside as he ate his breakfast that Monday morning in December. He decided right then to skip school and do a little rabbit hunting. The rabbits would be easy to track in the snow.

His expectations of a successful hunt were met by 11 AM, when he headed back toward the house with six rabbits in the game pouch of his hunting coat. That heavy backpack was starting to eat into his shoulders, and it was soon time for lunch. The thorn bush scratches on his legs were also an irritation, and he longed for a warm shower.

In the woodshed he emptied his game pouch and noted that one of the animals had bled extensively. He put on rubber gloves, cleaned the animals, and entered the house to shower before lunch. While undressing he noticed some rabbit blood stains on the tail of his shirt and the back of his undershorts. This meant he would have to put a new plastic liner in his game pouch.

For lunch he grabbed a quick glass of milk, some fresh cheese and crackers, and a piece of yesterday's apple pie. The farmer next door had made the cheese from a blend of goat's and cow's milk from his own herds. The cheese was especially tasty, so Bobby Jack had several pieces before he hurried off to his afternoon classes. He knew his mother would have fried rabbit for his dinner that night.

On Friday, Bobby Jack felt too ill to attend school. He was feverish and had a headache, some muscle pain, and a general ill feeling. When this continued until the next Friday, his mother insisted that he see the family physician. At that time, the following data were obtained:

Temperature	100.5°F
Pulse	68
Respirations	16
Blood pressure	128/88 mm Hg
White blood cell count	$10{,}800/mm^3$
Differential	Normal

A slight inguinal lymphadenopathy was present, but no other physical findings of significance were noted. There were several healed scratches on Bobby Jack's legs. Bobby Jack's physician was uncertain of the diagnosis and decided to hospitalize his patient. Blood was collected for culture and serologic testing.

Two days later, after symptomatic therapy, Bobby Jack was given an intensive physical examination, at which time a small ulcer was noted under his left buttock. At this time the clinical bacteriology laboratory reported that they had not yet isolated any suspected pathogen from the blood culture. They reminded the physician that they would need another serum sample before agglutination tests would be meaningful.

Questions

1. What three possible diseases are suggested by Bobby Jack's immediate past history?
2. What zoonoses are associated with rabbits?
3. What zoonoses are associated with milk and milk products?
4. Is any disease suggested by scratches from thorny bushes?
5. Is it expected that a blood culture would still be negative after 2 days of incubation? Explain.
6. What will the blood culture reveal if this is a case of tularemia? Of listeriosis?
7. What special culture conditions are needed for the bacteriologic diagnosis of tularemia? Of listeriosis?
8. Many laboratories do not attempt to isolate the agent of tularemia. Why?
9. What serologic test(s) would the clinical laboratory plan to use in this case?
10. What can be concluded from serologic tests in the absence of a second serum sample?

11. What are the expected results of serologic testing when acute and convalescent serum samples are available?
12. Can strain differences account for the semichronicity of this case?

Student Questions

Case 2 A Food-Borne Zoonosis

Maria Alvarado was in her seventh month of pregnancy and was making every effort to follow her doctor's orders to eat a well-balanced diet each day. Fortunately, where she lived near Los Angeles, it was easy to find fresh fruit and vegetables all year around. Mexican-style rice and refried beans fulfilled the cereal and part of the protein requirement. Fortunately, Maria loved cheese, and her doctor said at last week's visit that she should use it even more generously with her tacos, enchiladas, and other dishes.

But eating so much cheese was discomforting to Maria. Her complaint of constipation faded, however, as she developed flu-like symptoms. Fever, chills, and a more serious back pain did not diminish over a 5-day period. Suddenly she began premature contractions and was rushed to the hospital by her son, Ricardo, where she delivered a daughter. The infant was obviously weak, quickly developed circulatory and respiratory problems, and died the next day. The Alvarado family denied authorization for an autopsy on religious grounds.

Blood cultures and vaginal swabs were collected from Maria immediately after delivery. Several colonies resembling beta-hemolytic streptococci were recovered from the blood culture 24 hours later. Only one or two colonies of beta-hemolytic organisms were recovered from the vaginal swabs.

Questions

1. This is clearly a case of maternal-fetal transmission of a disease. Name five diseases that are transplacentally transmitted.
2. What are the major pathologic and microbiologic findings expected in the infant?

3. Maria had only a flu-like illness. Is this typical of the pathogen in this case?
4. Blood cultures revealed colonies resembling beta-hemolytic streptococci. Is it highly probable that *Streptococcus pyogenes* or group B streptococci caused this disease?
5. What is cold enrichment? Would it have been useful for blood cultures? For vaginal swab cultures?
6. Are special serotypes of this pathogen associated with human disease? Or special phage types? Explain.
7. What was the original source of the pathogen?
8. What are the expectations that an epidemic of infections by this agent will develop?
9. What public health measures are used to control the source and spread of this disease?
10. Is there a racial tendency to develop this disease?
11. Is there a sexual selection of this disease?
12. What immunologically depressed conditions favor this illness?
13. What are the usual manifestations of this disease in adults?
14. How does this pathogen escape the immune system of the human host?

Student Questions

Case 3 A Child's Farm Visit

Dane M., a 5-year-old city dweller, was especially happy to spend 2 weeks on his grandparents' dairy farm. He would get to see Grandpa milk the cows, help feed the chickens and gather eggs, play with the kittens and cats in the dairy barns, and ride the new pony Grandpa had bought for him. One of Dane's favorite play areas was under the milk shed, where he, the cats, and their kittens could escape the summer heat.

On the last day of his visit, Grandma noted several red spots on the back of Dane's thigh and was thus not terribly surprised when her daughter called the next day to report that Dane had been scratching those spots because they itched so much. Dane's mother said that some of those erythematous areas had little blisters near their center. Two days later, serpent-like tracks were seen to radiate from a few of these lesions. This frightened Dane's mother, so she called her pediatrician for an appointment.

Questions

1. Is this disease treatable? How?
2. Plumbers, construction workers, and house repairmen are adults who may contract this disease. How and where is this disease acquired? Is it restricted to farm settings?
3. What changes from normal would you expect in the white blood cell count?
4. Does this disease have a single etiology? Explain.
5. What is the most common etiologic agent?
6. Why is the disease so superficial in appearance?
7. This type of disease can be acquired by swimmers, yet is not called swimmer's itch. Explain.
8. Is this a dermal manifestation of a more serious systemic disease? Explain.

Student Questions

Case 4 It's From the Birds

Carl M., a 41-year-old employee in a turkey processing plant, became ill only 10 days after coming on the job. He worked on the receiving dock. Here the birds were taken from the cages, their legs were banded together, and they were placed on a moving conveyor that carried them into the building. Carl didn't feel terribly ill at first but had a slight headache, a more noticeable backache, which he first attributed to the bending and lifting required on his job, and a slight cough. In the following days, his cough became more persistent but seldom produced much sputum. He continued to develop other respiratory complaints—rapid breathing and dyspnea but no pleuritic pain.

On visiting his doctor's clinic, chest x-rays revealed consolidation in Carl's right lung. Since his illness had emerged gradually, his physician suspected avian tuber-

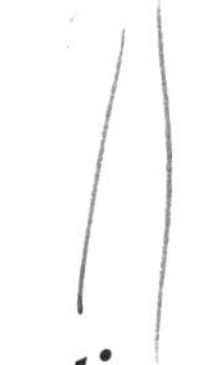

culosis and began treatment with streptomycin and isoniazid. After speaking to his wife about the diagnosis of tuberculosis and the failure of the doctor to perform a skin test or take cultures, Carl consulted a second physician. This physician made a different diagnosis and changed Carl's therapy.

Questions

1. Which zoonoses are anticipated to occur in a poultry processing plant?
2. Which of these are respiratory diseases?
3. This disease had a gradual onset. Does that eliminate certain zoonoses?
4. Is this gradual onset pathognomonic of avian tuberculosis?
5. If this were avian tuberculosis, was the initial therapy acceptable?
6. What other drugs could have been recommended?
7. What criteria eliminate anthrax as the likely diagnosis?
8. Turkeys are not psittacine birds, but could this be psittacosis (ornithosis)?
9. Describe the life cycle of the etiologic agent of psittacosis.
10. What is the meaning of the TWAR strain of ornithosis-causing bacteria?
11. What therapy would you, as the second physician, recommend?
12. What culture procedures should the first physician have requested to support his diagnosis?

Student Questions

Case 5 Taken from Tucson

David and Debra, successfully employed in their own boutique in a suburb of New York City, were pleased that their winter vacation had evolved just as planned. The Christmas season had reached a new sales high, and during the first part of January the weather had been simply horrible. But here they were at the end of January concluding their second week on a little ranch not far from Tucson. This was not a resort ranch; it was a working ranch with plenty of cattle, a few goats, and lots of chickens about. The temperature had been in the 70s every day, the sky was always clear and sun-filled, and their only complaint was a small dust storm on the day of their arrival. Now it was their last Sunday, time to pack the bags, head home, and make certain everything was in order for the Valentine's Day trade.

Monday in New York was a disaster. Both David and Debra woke up with bad headaches but attributed this to their long flight home. At work, both of them complained of feeling chilly but blamed it on the cold New York City weather. During the day, David began to feel progressively worse and at home that night found his temperature to be 101.5°F. Debra felt about the same as in the morning—headache and chilly. The couple both thought they had contracted the flu so didn't consult a doctor. After 2 or 3 more days, Debra began to feel almost normal again. Her fever never exceeded 99.7°F the entire time. During that time, David's condition had followed a different course. He had a higher, though not excessive fever, completely lost his appetite, and developed a dry cough and chest pain.

He felt too tired to work and stayed home in bed on Wednesday through Saturday. By Sunday and again on Monday he felt somewhat better. His cough and fever gradually disappeared, he regained his appetite and strength, and he was himself again after an illness of 2 weeks.

Questions

1. What are the prospects that David and Debra had the same illness?
2. If this is a zoonosis, which zoonoses are possible, and which can be ruled out?
3. Are horses, cattle, or other ranch animals implicated in this disease?
4. Why is the course of the disease so different in the two individuals?
5. What zoonoses are associated with Western ranch life? With apartment dwelling in New York City?
6. What features of their vacation or trip home are compatible with this disease?
7. What other respiratory diseases, nonzoonotic in origin, could mimic this disease?
8. What is the life cycle of nonbacterial pathogens that cause zoonotic respiratory disease?

Student Questions

Case 6 Christmas with the Family

Paul and his wife Cindy decided to spend the Christmas holidays on her parents' farm. Some good country cooking with the usual holiday dishes would be a real treat. It was a quiet time of the year for most farmers, and Paul anticipated several hours of leisure each day in front of the fireplace.

Cindy's father had other ideas, however. Paul's visit made it an opportune time for him to slaughter a pig. Help was needed to hoist the animal onto the slaughtering rack, grind the sausage, render the lard, and cook some pig skins. Besides, it would only take a couple of days, and then the "kids" could sleep till noon every day if they wished. Later there would be time for snowmobiling, ice-skating, and evenings in front of the fire.

Those 10 days in the country seemed even more enjoyable to Paul after he returned to work. The year-end inventory hadn't been completed, the tax forms had to be prepared for his employees, and plans had to be finalized for the end of January white sale. These problems, added to the daily routine, seemed to take their toll on Paul. What he thought on Monday was just a stress headache, if anything, got worse every day. By Wednesday, his back and knees were aching, and he decided to stay home from work. In the midst of a morning nap, he broke out in a heavy sweat that was soon followed by shaking chills. He thought the break in his fever signaled a recovery from the flu, or whatever it was, but that night his face felt hot and his temperature, earlier that day 100.4°F, was now 101°F.

On Thursday morning in his doctor's office, Paul still had a high temperature. His physical findings included a pronounced splenomegaly and enlarged cervical lymph nodes. Blood was drawn for blood cultures, and a clot tube was drawn for serologic studies. His doctor ruled out infectious mononucleosis, tularemia, influenza, and typhoid fever. He assured Paul that the diagnosis could be confirmed next week with further serologic testing and started him on antibiotics.

Questions

1. How could the physician eliminate infectious mononucleosis, tularemia, influenza, and typhoid fever?
2. What zoonoses are possible in midwinter in a rural setting?
3. Cindy never contracted this disease. Explain.
4. Would you expect Cindy's mother and father to develop this disease?
5. Special cultural conditions are sometimes needed for bacteriologic diagnoses. Prepare a table that summarizes these in relationship to zoonotic organisms.
6. What is meant by "febrile agglutinin" test?
7. Therapy for this disease is often necessary for several weeks. How does this relate to the nature of the infection?
8. What are the major side effects of long-term, broad-spectrum antibiotic therapy?

Student Questions

Case 7 Skip Day Sickness

Senior skip day had been a great success. For the first time in years the teachers never learned the magic date—June 2—a date that every senior at Dearborn High School would remember for a lifetime.

The day didn't really begin until 2 PM, when everyone gathered at the mall. Out of a class of 63 seniors, 47 showed up. The assignments had already been made. Paper plates, cups, and plastic knives and forks were purchased by the "service crew." The "hamburger crew" had the meat, buns, mustard, and ketchup under control. The "drinks crew" had plenty of canned pop but would need to stop for ice on the way out of town. A salad and baked beans were purchased at the deli, and the gang took off for Lakeside Country Park.

The softball game got under way immediately, and the Frisbee contest drew a lot of participants. The girls in the hamburger crew got the grills going, and soon everyone was occupied. Of course, the day would set a new high temperature record, and soon the pop supply was exhausted. Some members of the drinks crew set off for more ice and soda while the softball players sat about and complained of the heat. Finally one of them got the idea for a quick swim in the lake. The lakeshore was muddy, and the cleanest place to enter the water was just past the muskrat burrows on the dam. Although none of the girls would join them, the guys had fun cooling off in the water. When they heard the drinks crew drive in, they headed back to the picnic tables and another round of hamburgers and cold soda.

Principal Weaver was dismayed to learn that six senior boys were not at school on Monday a week later and wouldn't be at the rehearsal for the commencement exercise. The school nurse told him that the parents of all six had called in and described the same illness—a high fever, headache, muscle soreness, and a slight jaundice. At least a couple of the boys had upset stomachs and had vomited. Each was under the care of his own family physician. Principal Weaver thought it was strange that only some of the senior boys of the skip day crowd and none of the girls were ill.

Questions

1. What are the major clues in this case that lead one to the correct diagnosis?
2. Assume for a moment that this is a food-borne but not a zoonotic illness. What are the possible causes of such a disease?
3. Is the Jarisch-Herxheimer reaction a risk of treatment?
4. How does the pathogen in this case relate to other taxonomic groups of bacteria?
5. Describe the structure of the pathogen in this case, particularly as it is distinguished from closely related organisms.
6. What wild and domestic animals are common sources of the disease in this case?
7. How is this disease diagnosed?
8. This disease is not caused by a gram-positive organism, yet penicillin is the recommended therapeutic. Explain.
9. Describe the laboratory diagnosis of water-borne zoonoses.
10. What serologic procedures are used to diagnose this disease?

Student Questions

Case 8 Cat's Cradle

Tabby slept comfortably stretched out in his basket placed next to the hot air register. Even when the furnace fan kicked on, Tabby hardly moved. How cats could stand so much heat was a good problem for veterinary physiologists.

Everything wasn't this peaceful at the hospital. Tabby's owner, Gladys, had just delivered a preemie. The little boy weighed only 5 lb 4 oz and was 6 weeks premature. The child was taken to the intensive care nursery and after careful examination was thought to have an infectious disease. Among the symptoms leading to this conclusion were a rash, petechiae, a possible pneumonitis, and chorioretinitis. Spinal fluid and blood were collected to aid in the diagnosis. Unfortunately, the placenta had been discarded and was not available for study.

Questions

1. What infectious diseases are associated with chorioretinitis of the newborn?
2. What is the TORCH syndrome?
3. What diseases or agents mimic those of the TORCH group?
4. What serologic tests must be considered in this case?
5. Is it possible to monitor pregnant women for this infection by serologic tests?
6. Of what value is the spinal fluid specimen in this case?
7. What is the meaning of IgM in sera of newborn infants?
8. Is the blood specimen also to be used to culture the pathogen responsible for this disease?
9. What further symptoms of disease will this baby develop during infancy? Are any of these sequelae permanent?
10. Should the mother and child receive treatment? If so, with what?
11. How is the TORCH group of diseases prevented?
12. What populations other than the mother-fetus relationship are subject to infection by the animal parasite in the TORCH complex?

Student Questions

Review Questions

1. Which of the following is **not** a zoonosis?

   A. Anthrax
   B. Diphtheria
   C. Plague
   D. Salmonellosis
   E. Yersiniosis

2. Which of the following is often transmitted through eggs and poultry?

   A. Tuberculosis
   B. Listeriosis
   C. Brucellosis

D. Salmonellosis
E. All of the above

3. A principal source of hepatitis A infection is

A. Shellfish
B. Poultry
C. Undercooked pork
D. Eggs
E. Milk

4. Swimmer's itch is caused by

A. Excessive dryness of the skin from chlorinated water
B. Avian trematodes infecting a human host
C. A dermatophytic fungus
D. Partially attenuated herpes simplex virus
E. None of the above

5. Weil's disease is caused by

A. Contact with contaminated animal hair
B. Direct contact with human feces
C. *Leptospira interrogans*
D. The same agent that causes erysipeloid
E. *Toxocara canis*

6. Which of the following zoonoses is often expressed as a respiratory disease?

A. Rabies
B. Cryptosporidiosis
C. Echinococcosis
D. Salmonellosis
E. Q fever

7. Which of the following is caused by the "armed tapeworm"?

A. Schistosomiasis
B. Toxoplasmosis
C. Hookworm disease
D. Cysticercosis
E. Echinococcosis

8. The Widal test is

A. Useful in diagnosing Weil-Felix disease
B. An agglutination test
C. A dye exclusion test used to diagnose toxoplasmosis
D. Useful in diagnosing Weil's disease
E. A specific test for trichinosis

9. The trichina worm infection of humans

A. Is acquired from eating undercooked meat
B. Induces a pronounced eosinophilia

9 Arthropod-Borne Diseases

A special subdivision of the zoonoses treats only those zoonoses transmitted by arthropod vectors. Almost without exception the arthropod takes a blood meal from an infected animal reservoir and thereby acquires the pathogenic agent. The infectious agent may grow in its arthropod host, but even if this does not occur, the arthropod transfers the agent to the human host when taking another meal.

The phylum Arthropoda is divided into three classes. The class Crustacea contains few vectors of diseases found in the United States. In other parts of the world, they are important intermediaries in the life cycle of human pathogens. The class Arachnida includes ticks and mites, which are very important vectors of viral, rickettsial, and bacterial diseases. These diseases may be acquired from lower mammals or may be restricted to the human race. The class Insecta, which includes fleas, lice, and mosquitoes, transmits several important human diseases. Flies and bugs, also classified as insects, are often erroneously considered only as mechanical vectors, but they may also serve as biologic vectors.

Some arthropods are themselves liable to a lethal disease by the agent they transmit (lice—epidemic typhus), whereas others are entirely resistant and may pass the agent by transovarial transmission (ticks—Rocky Mountain spotted fever). Some vectors are an essential host for a maturation stage in the life cycle of the agent it transmits (mosquito—malaria). The human encounter with arthropods is in most instances accidental; nevertheless, the dense population achieved by these vectors at certain seasons of the year contributes to diseases that may occur in epidemic proportions.

A few of the arthropod-borne diseases may be transmitted by other means. Tularemia is transmissible by direct contact or ingestion. Plague, another example, is transmitted human to human as an airborne disease.

It is important to note the dominance of rickettsia and viruses in arthropod-borne diseases in the United States. This places a limitation on treatment of these diseases, since viral diseases seldom have a specific therapy. Several broad-spectrum antibiotics are effective in treating the rickettsioses. Penicillin derivatives are very effective against arthropod-transmitted spirochetoses.

Within the United States, ticks are a primary vector (Table 9-1), but due to the prevalence of malaria in other parts of the world, mosquitoes are the most important vector on a worldwide basis (Tables 9-2 and 9-3).

Table 9-1. Tick-borne diseases found in the United States

Disease	Etiologic agent	Type of agent	Major animal reservoir	Tick vectors
Babesiosis	*Babesia bovis*, *B. microti*, *B. divergens*	Protozoan	Cattle	*Ixodes* species, *Rhipicephalus* species
Colorado tick fever	Arbovirus	Virus	Squirrels, mice	*Dermacentor andersoni*
Ehrlichiosis	*Ehrlichia canis*	Rickettsia	Dogs	*Dermacentor variabilis* *Rhipicephalus* species
Lyme disease	*Borrelia burgdorferi*	Spirochete	Deer, field mice, other vertebrates	*Ixodes dammini* *Amblyomma americanum*
Relapsing fever	*Borrelia recurrentis*	Spirochete	Rodents	*Ornithodoros hermsi* *Ornithodoros turicata* (Louse-borne disease also occurs)
Rocky Mountain spotted fever	*Rickettsia rickettsii*	Rickettsia	Rabbits, squirrels	*Dermacentor andersoni* *Dermacenter variabilis* *Amblyomma americanum*
Tularemia	*Francisella tularensis*	Bacterium	Rabbits	*Dermacentor andersoni*

Solving the cases described in this chapter will rely on your knowledge of geography, seasonal influences on the arthropod population, habits of the arthropod, and of course aspects of the disease itself—unique lesion, incubation time, and so on.

Key Words and Phrases

It would be well to add the names of the arthropod vectors to this listing.

Antigenic variation in *Borrelia*
Arbovirus
Biologic vector
Blackwater fever
Brill's disease
Erythema chronicum migrans
Erythrocytic cycle
Eschar
Gametocytes
Horizontal transmission
Jarisch-Herxheimer reaction
Lyme disease
Mechanical vector
Merozoite
Proteus Ox-19, Ox-2, and Ox-K
Reservoir
Ring form
Schizont
Sentinel birds
Spirochetosis
Spotted fever group
Sylvatic plague
Typhus group
Vector
Vertical transmission
Weil-Felix test

Table 9-2. Arthropod-borne diseases rarely found in the United States

Disease	Etiologic agent	Type of agent	Animal reservoir	Vector	Types of vector
Dengue	Dengue virus (*Flavivirus*)	Viral	Humans	*Aedes* species	Mosquito
Filariasis	*Wuchereria* and *Brugia*	Nematode	Humans	*Aedes*, *Anopheles*, *Culex*, other genera	Mosquito
Leishmaniasis	*Leishmania donovani*, *L. braziliensis*, and others	Protozoan	Humans	*Phlebotomus* and *Lutzomyia*	Sandfly
Loiasis	*Loa loa*	Nematode	Humans	*Chrysops*	Deer flies
Malaria	*Plasmodium vivax*, *P. falciparum*, and others	Protozoan	Humans	*Anopheles* species	Mosquito
Onchocerciasis	*Onchocerca volvulus*	Nematode	Humans	*Simulium*	Black flies
Scrub typhus	*Rickettsia tsutsugamushi*	Rickettsia	Humans	*Leptotrombidium* species	Mite
Trypanosomiasis	*Trypanosoma rhodesiense*, *T. gambiense*, and others	Protozoan	Antelope	*Glossina dorsalis*	Tsetse fly
Yellow fever	*Flavivirus*	Viral	Humans, monkey	*Aedes*	Mosquito

Table 9-3. Arthropod-borne diseases sometimes found in the United States

Disease	Etiologic agent	Type of agent	Animal reservoir	Vector	Type of vector
California encephalitis	Bunyavirus	Viral	Small mammals	*Aedes*	Mosquito
Chagas' disease	*Trypanosoma cruzi*	Protozoan	Opossum, armadillo	*Triatoma* (reduviid) bug	Bug
Encephalitis	St. Louis, Eastern, and Western equine encephalitis arbovirus (*Flavivirus*)	Viral	Birds	*Culex* species	Mosquito
Endemic typhus	*Rickettsia typhi*	Rickettsia	Small mammals	*Xenopsylla* and other fleas	Flea
Epidemic typhus	*Rickettsia prowazekii*	Rickettsia	Humans, small mammals	*Pediculus humanus*	Louse
Plague	*Yersinia pestis*	Bacterium	Rat, wild rodents	*Xenopsylla cheopis*	Flea
Relapsing fever	*Borrelia hermsii*	Spirochete	Humans	*Pediculus humanus*	Louse
Rickettsialpox	*Rickettsia akari*	Rickettsia	Mice	*Allodermanyssus sanguineus*	Mite
Trench fever	*Rochalimaea quintana*	Rickettsia	Humans	*Pediculus humanus*	Louse

Abbreviations

EEE
RMSF
SLE
VEE
WEE

Information Sources

Brenner, R.R., and de la Merced Stoka, A., editors: Chagas' disease vectors, CRC Press, Inc., 1987, Boca Raton.

Burgdorfer, W., and Anacker, R.L., editors: Rickettsiae and rickettsial diseases, Academic Press, Inc., 1981, New York.

Butler, T.: Plague and other *Yersinia* infections, Plenum Press, 1983, New York.

Dengue haemorrhagic fever: diagnosis, treatment and control, WHO, 1986, Geneva.

Goddard, J.: A physician's guide to arthropods of medical importance, CRC Press, Inc., 1993, Boca Raton.

Harden, V.A.: Rocky Mountain spotted fever: history of a twentieth-century disease, Johns Hopkins University Press, 1990, Baltimore.

Hubbert, W.T., McCulloch, W.F., and Schnurrenberger, R.P., editors: Diseases transmitted from animals to man, edition 6, C.C. Thomas, 1975, Springfield, IL.

Kreier, J.P., editor: Malaria, Academic Press, Inc., 1980, New York.

Schlesinger, S., and Schlesinger, M.J.: Togaviridae and Flaviviridae, Liss, 1986, New York.

Steele, J.H., editor: CRC Handbook Series in Zoonosis, CRC Press, Inc., 1979, Boca Raton.

Tizard, I., editor: Immunology and pathogenesis of trypanosomiasis, CRC Press, Inc., 1985, Boca Raton.

Walker, D.H.: Biology of rickettsial diseases, vol. 1 and 2, CRC Press, Inc., 1988, Boca Raton.

Wilson, M.E.: A world guide to infections: diseases, distribution, diagnosis, Oxford University Press, 1991, Oxford.

Case 1 Scout Troop 116

Jon W., an Eagle Scout in Troop 116 of Hershey, Pennsylvania, was about to miss his first troop meeting after 4 years of perfect attendance. The troop had enjoyed perfect weather during their spring camp-out the previous weekend. That was the troop's last activity prior to the awards ceremony scheduled for Friday. Jon made the camping trip but would miss the awards ceremony.

Jon's mother had phoned the troop leader with the news that Jon had a severe headache, was feverish, and for a boy in good physical condition was complaining a lot about aches and pains in his back. She said that Jon had a slight rash on the palms of his hands and that she was taking him to the family doctor. He would have to miss the troop meeting and maybe even a few days of school next week.

Questions

1. Does the development of this case in Pennsylvania eliminate certain etiologies?
2. How does the season of the year influence a physician's approach to an unexplained rash?
3. What insect-transmitted disease is characterized by an early rash on the palms and the other symptoms mentioned?
4. What insect-transmitted diseases should be considered here?
5. Is the time between the scout troop camp-out and Jon's illness consistent with an infectious etiology?
6. Can this disease be transmitted person to person?
7. How do insects transmit diseases to humans? To their offspring?
8. Is arthritis or other sequelae associated with this illness?
9. Why aren't campers immunized against this disease?
10. Is the Weil-Felix test applicable here?
11. What is the basis of the Weil-Felix test?
12. What therapeutic options exist for this disease?
13. Is any therapy contraindicated?
14. What is the prognosis in the absence of effective therapy?
15. Is this disease communicated person to person?

Student Questions

Case 2 Romance by the Riverside

Richard and Elaine started dating during the winter of their senior year in high school. After graduation, Richard worked during the summer on the family ranch, Loma del Rio. Elaine enrolled for summer school at San Diego State College. It was an easy drive from her home to the campus each day, and she wanted to pick up some credit hours so she would have a lighter schedule during her freshman year.

During the summer, the couple saw each other every weekend. Sometimes it was just to watch TV, rent a movie, or take a walk along the small stream that flowed through the ranch. During one of these walks in late July, on an especially warm night, the couple went "skinny-dipping" in a section of the stream that had been dammed to form a small pond.

When Elaine called Richard the next Friday to arrange their weekend plans, she was surprised to learn that he had not worked that day. This was unusual because the migrant Mexican workers who had been at the ranch all summer had left just the week before and Richard's father needed the help. But Richard apparently had a virus infection—headache, some fever, and vague muscle aches and pains. During Saturday and Sunday, Richard's condition remained much the same, but then he began to develop joint and chest pains. On Tuesday, Richard had a violent chill, appeared cyanotic, and an hour later spiked a fever of 104°F. When he became delirious and vomited, he was rushed to the hospital, where the diagnosis of his disease was quickly determined.

Questions

1. Are there unique summertime fevers found in Southern California?
2. Do employment and outdoor labor on a ranch near San Diego suggest any particular infection?
3. Could Richard have a sexually transmitted disease?
4. Could Richard's illness be related to nighttime skinny-dipping?
5. Could Richard's Mexican coworkers have directly transmitted some unusual disease to him?
6. What infectious diseases can you think of that are common in Mexico, but not in the United States, that could be brought here by migrant laborers?
7. Which of the diseases suggested from question 6 are diagnosed by an examination of blood or tissue smears?
8. Are Richard's symptoms compatible with any of these diseases?
9. Describe the etiologic agent and the life cycle of pathogens you listed as your answer to question 6.
10. Are the "correct" mosquitoes for the transmission of malaria found in the United States? If so, why isn't malaria endemic in the United States?
11. How is malaria diagnosed?
12. How is malaria treated? Describe drug resistance as it applies to malaria.
13. What is cryptic malaria?
14. What is blackwater fever?

Student Questions

Case 3 Tick-Borne Disease

It was a foggy and damp spring morning, but Jim was determined to look for mushrooms. An hour later, dressed in heavy trousers, a sweatshirt, and a rain hat, he was tramping through the woods. Later, with nothing to show for his time, Jim was at his car ready to head home.

At home he threw his damp clothes over a chair and showered in the unfinished basement bathroom. He examined himself closely for ticks but found none.

By the next evening the weather, though cool, had cleared. When Bob called to suggest they go fishing, it was only moments until Jim was in the basement readying his fishing gear. He put on the old clothes he had worn mushroom hunting the day before and was ready to go when he heard Bob's car horn.

It was 10 PM when they got back to town and 10:45 by the time they had cleaned the fish and congratulated themselves on their good luck. Jim was tired; he washed his hands and face and went to bed. The next morning he showered and began to dry himself when he noticed a small tick, which he removed from his right shoulder.

Exactly 14 days later, again in the shower, Jim noticed an erythematous circle about 4 cm in diameter in the exact area where he had found the tick. The very center of the red area had a faint purplish color. By 9:30 AM Jim was in his doctor's waiting room with his self-made diagnosis well in mind.

Questions

1. What tick-borne diseases are common in the spring?
2. Which of these are bacterial diseases, and which are rickettsial diseases?
3. Jim never had a complaint of headache, fever, malaise, or other symptoms so common in infectious disease. Does this suggest or eliminate any specific tick-borne disease(s)?
4. What key feature of this disease allowed Jim to make his own diagnosis?
5. What spirochetal diseases are transmitted by ticks in the United States?
6. Compare spirochetes with other curved bacterial forms.

7. Why is effective therapy so important in this disease?
8. How is the diagnosis definitely established?
9. What is/are the major reservoir(s) of the pathogen in this case?
10. This is only recently a reportable disease. How do you account for this in relation to your answer to question 7?

Student Questions

Case 4 A Family Vacation

John L., age 62, had taken early retirement and had enjoyed a quiet winter at home. His daily nap in front of the fireplace made him the target of regular teasing from his wife. To prove he was still young at heart, John organized a spring outing for the entire family at Grand Canyon National Park. John, his wife, their two children, Marla (age 32) and Mark (age 35), and their two spouses made the trip. They spent a full week hiking through the canyon trails, sleeping in the park cabins at night.

About 10 days after their return home and within 2 days of each other, all six family members developed a fever, chills, an excruciating headache, and muscle aches and pains. About the time Mark and his wife (the first two to become ill) decided to give up on aspirin as a self-cure and call their doctor, they began to feel much better. They told the other family members that they would be well in a day or two, and this seemed to be the case.

This was a short-lived recovery, however, as within 3 days the illness struck Mark and his wife again with another bout of fever, heavy sweating, chills, and headache. At this time, both of them were examined by their doctor. The following findings for Mark were not that much different from the data found for his wife.

Blood pressure	112/78 mm Hg
Temperature	99°F (37°C)
Respirations	20
Pulse	96

Complaint: Sore muscles, strong headache, fever, and chills 3 days ago that disappeared and returned today

Physical examination: No remarkable findings

Hematology report: Thrombocytopenia, leukocytosis

Spinal fluid report: Neutrophilic pleocytosis

Questions

1. What infectious diseases are characterized by intermittent bouts of severe fever and chills with an accompanying headache?
2. Which of these diseases are found in the United States?
3. Which of these diseases could be associated with hiking and camping in an arid region of the United States?
4. What zoonotic reservoirs are suspected in this situation?
5. What vectors are suspected in this case?
6. Is the failure of all six individuals to notice any vector suggestive of any specific vector or disease?
7. What evidence, if any, suggests a rickettsial disease?
8. What evidence, if any, suggests a spirochetal etiology?
9. What are the etiologic agents of nonvenereal spirochetal diseases in the United States?
10. What is the basis for the diagnosis of endemic typhus?
11. What is the basis for the diagnosis of relapsing fever?
12. What symptoms would be expected if this were a case of sylvatic plague?
13. If this is a tick-borne disease, why did no one notice a tick or tick bite?
14. What antibiotics could logically be chosen for treatment of these cases?
15. Is the Jarisch-Herxheimer reaction a possibility if intensive, successful therapy is applied?
16. What is the pathophysiologic etiology of the Jarisch-Herxheimer reaction?
17. What treatment is recommended to prevent other hiker-campers from contracting this disease?
18. How do the two waves of fever and chills relate to the genetic versatility of the pathogen?

Student Questions

Case 5 Hurricane Aftermath

The volunteer medical unit from Metropolitan Hospital did not go in immediately after the hurricane. The first units to provide medical assistance after the storm struck the island were military groups, including army, navy, and national guard. Only 2 weeks later did the governor allow civilian volunteer groups on the island.

Kathy Halstead was a nurse in this first civilian group. What she saw in the rural areas of the island would make a lifelong memory—devastated buildings, upturned trees, flooded roads and fields everywhere. Although she had an abundant supply of insect repellent, the mosquitoes and little black no-see-ums seemed to have enough intelligence to wait until Kathy's neck, arms, and legs were washed in sweat before they came for their blood meal. Although this had the appearance of a glamour trip, Kathy was glad when their 10-day tour ended and she could return to the comforts of life in Indianapolis.

Unfortunately, it didn't turn out that way. Two days after resuming her work at Metropolitan Hospital, she developed a severe headache, her fever was an alarming 102.2°F, she felt nauseous, and she vomited before she could see Dr. Bruce Phelps. Bruce had been a part of the civilian medical relief team on the island and was pretty certain what caused Kathy's illness. He took a blood sample for a hematocrit determination and platelet count and drew a clot tube for an acute serum serologic test. He prescribed acetaminophen for fever control and told Kathy to observe herself carefully for any petechia, nosebleed, or other bleeding that might develop during the night. Kathy stayed in the hospital for 3 days. Seventeen days later a serum sample evaluated against the acute sample confirmed the diagnosis.

Questions

1. What arthropod-borne diseases are associated with the Caribbean islands?
2. Which of these are mosquito-borne?
3. Which of these are no-see-um (sandfly)–borne?
4. Are mosquitoes or sandflies capable of transovarial transmission of infectious agents?
5. Aren't severe headache and elevated fever typical of all arthropod-borne diseases?
6. What is the reason for the hematocrit and platelet studies in this case?
7. Is there a special reason for the acetaminophen rather than another agent to control Kathy's fever?
8. Is a 17-day interval appropriate for acute and convalescent serum sampling?
9. What serologic test(s) is/are appropriate for diagnosing this case?
10. Where do tissue culture techniques enter into the diagnosis of arthropod-borne diseases?
11. Does this disease exist in the continental 48 states?
12. Is your answer to question 11 related to vector availability in the continental 48 states?

Student Questions

Case 6 Summer Encephalitis

Joan, a 12-year-old schoolgirl, had never traveled much from the rural county in Kansas where she had been born, but when her cousin Kim invited her to spend part of the summer vacation in Houston, her parents said, "Why not?" On June 12, her parents began the journey down the interstate with the plan to take in a baseball game in Dallas, where they would spend the weekend before continuing on to Houston.

On June 16, as the family neared the outskirts of Houston, a local news report coming over the car radio alerted listeners to an outbreak of encephalitis in the city. A physician interviewed on the program stated his opinion that unusual heavy rainfall that spring had increased the mosquito population far above normal. He hypothesized that the six cases of encephalitis now in Houston hospitals would prove to have St. Louis encephalitis virus as its cause. Just as Joan's father pulled into a gas station, she heard the physician mention something about sentinel chickens being used to determine the cause of the encephalitis. Unfortunately, when he turned off the motor, the radio went dead and Joan couldn't hear the rest of the interview.

Questions

1. What is the geographic distribution of St. Louis encephalitis?
2. Is the distribution of St. Louis encephalitis dependent on its transmission by a certain vector?
3. What is the relationship of the St. Louis encephalitis virus to other encephalitogenic viruses?
4. Are all encephalitic viruses transmitted by the same vector?
5. How is St. Louis encephalitis related, if at all, to sleeping sickness in horses; that is, are horses the natural reservoir of this virus?
6. Are birds a reservoir of St. Louis encephalitis?
7. What are sentinel chickens, and how are they used to monitor viral encephalitis?

8. What does the term *arbovirus* mean? Is it a family name? A genus name?
9. What is Joan's risk of getting St. Louis encephalitis while in Houston? Is it probable that her cousin Kim is already immune to it?
10. What are the major risk factors for contracting St. Louis encephalitis as opposed to a tick-borne disease?

Student Questions

Review Questions

1. Epidemic typhus is transmitted by
   A. The body louse
   B. Mites
   C. *Culex* mosquitoes
   D. *Anopheles* mosquitoes
   E. Ticks
2. The clinical symptoms of malaria are due to
   A. The erythrocytic cycle
   B. The exoerythrocytic cycle
   C. The paraerythrocytic cycle
   D. The paraexoerythrocytic cycle
   E. The sporozoites
3. A zoonotic febrile illness characterized by a distinctive skin lesion in the early phase and joint pains in the later phase of the disease could easily be
   A. Lyme disease
   B. Q fever
   C. Relapsing fever
   D. Syphilis
   E. Typhus

4. Which of the following pairs of arthropod vector and disease is **not** correct?
   A. Rat flea—endemic typhus
   B. Body louse—Brill's disease
   C. Dog tick—Rocky Mountain spotted fever
   D. House mouse mite—rickettsialpox
   E. Body louse—epidemic typhus

5. Which of the following diseases is **not** caused by a rickettsia?
   A. Relapsing fever
   B. Trench fever
   C. Ehrlichiosis
   D. Rickettsialpox
   E. Endemic typhus

6. The agglutination of special strains of *Proteus* bacteria may be useful in the diagnosis of
   A. Dengue
   B. Lyme disease
   C. Rocky Mountain spotted fever
   D. Colorado tick fever
   E. Tularemia

7. Which of the following zoonotic diseases is most common in the south central Atlantic seaboard states?
   A. Dengue
   B. Rocky Mountain spotted fever
   C. Scrub typhus
   D. Rickettsialpox
   E. Relapsing fever

8. Which of the following is **not** a matched pair?
   A. Blackwater fever—protozoan
   B. Erythema chronicum migrans—tick-borne disease
   C. Brill's disease—viral etiology
   D. Weil-Felix test—rickettsia
   E. Jarisch-Herxheimer reaction—therapy of a spirochetosis

9. Which of the following tropical diseases is typically transmitted by mosquitoes?
   A. Yellow fever
   B. Trypanosomiasis
   C. Scrub typhus
   D. Onchocerciasis
   E. Chagas' disease

10. Birds are the animal reservoir of
    A. Yellow fever
    B. St. Louis encephalitis

C. California encephalitis
D. Colorado tick fever
E. Ehrlichiosis

11. Transovarial transmission in ticks occurs in

A. Rocky Mountain spotted fever
B. Plague
C. Chagas' disease
D. Onchocerciasis
E. Scrub typhus

12. Which of the following zoonoses is the most easily transmitted person to person by nonarthropod means?

A. Rocky Mountain spotted fever
B. Plague
C. Malaria
D. Tularemia
E. Relapsing fever

10 Miscellaneous Infections

With the experience given by the earlier chapters to draw on, many of the cases presented here may be less of a challenge than expected. This is only true for some of the cases, of course. Not only do the cases here represent examples from bacteriology, virology, parasitology, and mycology, but also some of the cases quite honestly are rare, obscure examples of the extremes of infectious disease. These will provide the challenge and, when met, the feeling of accomplishment.

Key Words and Phrases

The previous word and phrase listings apply to this chapter.

Information Sources

See also Chapter 1 for additional references.

Brown, W.H., and Neva, F.A.: Basic clinical parasitology, edition 5, Appleton-Century-Crofts, Inc., 1983, New York.

Campbell, W.C., and Rew, R.S., editors: Chemotherapy of parasitic diseases, Plenum Press, 1986, New York.

Dubey, J.P.: Toxoplasmoses of animals and man, CRC Press, 1988, Boca Raton.

Gerety, R.J., editor: Hepatitis B, Academic Press, Inc., 1985, Orlando.

Grist, N.R., et al.: Diseases of infection, edition 2, Oxford University Press, 1993, Oxford.

Hoaglund, R.J.: Infectious mononucleosis, Grune & Stratton, 1967, New York.

Hollinger, F.B., et al.: Viral hepatitis, Raven Press, Inc., 1991, New York.

Markell, E.K., Voge, M.J., and John, D.T: Medical parasitology, edition 6, W.B. Saunders Co., 1986, Philadelphia.

Thompson, R.C.A., editor: The biology of echinococcosis and hydatid disease, Allen and Unwin, 1986, London.

Walls, K.W., and Schantz, P.M., editors: Immunodiagnosis of parasitic diseases, Academic Press, Inc., 1986, Orlando.

Warnock, D.W., and Richardson, M.D., editors: Fungal infection in the compromised host, John Wiley & Sons, Ltd., 1991, Chichester.

Case 1 The Bride's Banquet

Khanita was pleased with her new husband, obviously a man of means. He had flown to Saigon from Omaha to ask Khanita's parents to bless their wedding. Wisely, he had taken them expensive gifts and showed them a VCR tape of the home he was having built for his bride.

On his return from Saigon he had arranged all aspects of their wedding, a civil ceremony that would be followed by a religious ceremony when they visited their homeland later. He had planned a great feast for nearly 200 guests, most of them refugees from their war-torn country. The noodles, rice, spiced pork meat, tropical fruits, and other dishes were all delicious reminders of their earlier home abroad.

A week later in Honolulu, while on their way to Saigon, Khanita called one of her friends in Omaha. The woman was not at home, and her answering machine had the message that she would return from the doctor's office about 4 PM. That evening Khanita was able to complete her call but heard some disturbing news. Nearly 120 of her wedding guests had become ill with what seemed like an identical illness. Most of them had a low-grade fever, myalgia, and an unusual edema around their eyes. A few had a touch of diarrhea. After the diagnosis had been correctly made on the first of them who had visited the doctor, the call went out that eventually identified the disease among nearly two-thirds of the wedding guests. Khanita's friend said that even though the doctors knew what the disease was they weren't giving them any antibiotics or other prescription medicine.

Questions

1. What are the major clues in this vignette to a diagnosis?
2. Is this an infectious disease transmitted from a wedding guest to others in attendance?
3. What is the apparent incubation time of this disease?
4. Does the incubation time exclude most food-borne intoxications and infections?
5. What patient symptoms are most valuable in establishing the diagnosis?
6. What is the reservoir of this illness?
7. What measures are essential to prevent this disease?
8. Are there both domestic and natural reservoirs?
9. How is this disease diagnosed?
10. How is this disease treated, if at all?

Student Questions

Case 2 Desert Storm

Private Donatelli of the 7th Battalion Military Police unit was happy to have a night off-duty. Since the end of the Desert Storm campaign, he had been assigned to a Saudi unit guarding POWs. Now that the war was ended, they would soon be shipping these prisoners home. That could only mean that he would soon be going home too. This was his first night off since the cease fire and a good night for something special.

He decided to test his language skills by eating in a portable tent restaurant an enterprising local merchant had erected outside the military compound. As he struggled through a list of several foods whose names he remembered, Donatelli saw that he wasn't getting through to the cafe manager. The manager nodded his head, smiled, and then turned to his wife in the kitchen area of the tent. Within moments she was at his table with all manner of foods and beverages. Most of them tasted a little strange except the ground meat wrapped in grape leaves, which reminded him a little of the Italian meatballs his mother used to make.

When Donatelli finished his meal, the cafe owner refused any payment and sent the diner on his way. The next morning Donatelli felt a little dizzy when he climbed out of his cot. During the day he felt tired and thought the desert air had finally gotten to him, his mouth felt so dry. By evening he noticed he was having trouble focusing his eyes. The bright lights around the prison perimeter were killing his eyes. He told his sergeant that he was turning himself in to the medical unit.

Questions

1. Does this illness resemble any known "desert fever"?
2. Could incidental contact with louse-infested prisoners account for Private Donatelli's illness?
3. Do these symptoms resemble nerve gas poisoning?
4. Which of Private Donatelli's symptoms are most revealing of his illness?
5. Why don't other prison guards or prisoners have this illness?
6. Do you think the cafe owner and his wife have or will have this illness? Explain.
7. What microbial disease(s) would you consider?
8. Which of these diseases are infections, and which are intoxications?
9. Is this disease related to infant botulism? If so, how?
10. Is infant or adult botulism caused by a single bacterial agent or toxin? Explain.

Student Questions

Case 3 The Traveler

Howard was a 50-year-old executive of a United States shoe manufacturing company who had been to Uruguay several times in the past 3 years to sign contracts for hides and for a few speciality shoe designs. He enjoyed the grilled meats—beef, lamb, and occasionally pork—that one could get in restaurants in every village.

About a year before his present visit to his doctor, he began to have some dull pain in the margin of his chest and the upper segment of his abdomen. Medical examinations conducted at that time were not revealing. These pains were irregular and temporarily disappeared, only to return last month.

On examination at this time, Howard had the following vital signs:

Temperature	98.6°F
Pulse	72
Respirations	18
Blood pressure	140/82 mm Hg

Urinalysis was normal, and blood studies were normal with the possible exception of a slight eosinophilia (eosinophils 6%). The presence of an enlarged liver below the costal margin was the only abnormality. Chest x-ray and abdominal and chest ultrasonography were ordered. A heavily marginated cyst approximately 3.5 cm in diameter was observed in the liver. Chest films were normal.

Questions

1. What diseases found in Uruguay, and seldom encountered by persons remaining in the United States, are suggested by this history?
2. Describe the life cycle of the possible pathogen.
3. What features of this pathogen, including its disease process in humans, make this a difficult disease to eradicate?
4. Is it possible to use chemical sterilants before surgery to remove or drain the lesion?
5. Is there a useful skin test to aid in the diagnosis of this disease? Describe its preparation and use.
6. In what parts or regions of the world, other than Uruguay, does this disease exist?
7. Discuss serologic tests used in the diagnosis of this disease.

Student Questions

C. Is diagnosed by the examination of muscle biopsy
D. Is characterized by periorbital edema
E. All of the above

10. Rabies

A. Can be prevented by immunization with an attenuated virus vaccine
B. Is invariably fatal
C. Has a short incubation period of 3 to 5 days
D. Virus produces diagnostic Negri bodies in the brain of all rabid animals
E. Is transmissible only via animal bites

Case 4 A Real Shock

Peter H. was received in the emergency department as a transfer patient from a neighboring hospital, where he had an appendectomy 7 days previously. He recovered from the surgery without incident and was discharged. On the morning of the present day, he developed a headache and vomited twice after breakfast. He soon noted an erythematous rash on his chest. His wife returned him to the primary hospital, where he was noted to be disoriented and to have a fever of 102.5°F and a falling blood pressure. When he was later received at University Hospital, these findings were confirmed, his blood pressure now 78/48 mm Hg. In view of the critical state of the patient, the emergency physician opened the appendectomy scar, aspirated approximately 4 ml of pus, and initiated therapy with vancomycin. The specimen was sent to the laboratory for culture. Three days later Peter felt nearly normal except for a slight myalgia and muscle weakness. He was discharged the following day.

Questions

1. The rapid onset of this disease suggests toxin-producing organisms. Which do you suspect?
2. Describe the toxins potentially involved.
3. This began as a surgical procedure. What population of bacteria would you anticipate recovering from the pus in the abscess?
4. What culture procedures and results would be expected for this specimen?
5. Why was vancomycin selected for therapy rather than some other antibiotic?
6. What is the risk of this disease in the female population?
7. Is this disease a typical hospital-acquired infection or more often community-acquired?
8. What was the probable source of this infection—the surgeon, the patient himself, or other sources?

Student Questions

Case 5 The Tabernacle Church of the Unholy Visitation

Reverend Gutemann asked his congregation to gather for a special prayer meeting on Friday. After the regular Wednesday night meeting, he had learned that a second child in his congregation had died. This brought the death total to seven among the congregations in this part of West Virginia, Kentucky, and Tennessee. A state public health officer told Reverend Gutemann that nearly 600 members of this religious group in Appalachia were or had been ill. He further stated that he had court authorization to order medical treatment and immunization for all members of this religious order and that he was recommending a second immunization for all children in addition to their primary immunization, since numerous breaks in vaccine-induced immunity had occurred. He asked Reverend Gutemann if he had read or heard of several colleges closing for short periods of time due to outbreaks of this disease.

Reverend Gutemann began to develop his theme for the special Friday prayer session. He remembered an earlier epidemic like this 10 years ago that had been stopped by prayer and fasting before a court order could be issued to force them to vaccinate against God's will. He even remembered the health officer at that time telling about Koplik's spots and how that was the identifying mark of the disease.

Questions

1. What disease is diagnosed in part through the presence of Koplik's spots?
2. What are Koplik's spots?
3. What is the microbial etiology of this disease?
4. What are the major characteristics of this agent?
5. What are the major characteristics of other closely related pathogens?
6. Discuss the vaccine for this disease, its nature, and its use.
7. Is this vaccine similar to the vaccine for other members of this etiologic group?
8. This disease is normally quite mild. Is it cost-effective to require two immunizations to provide immunity against this disease?
9. How is this disease related to subacute sclerosing panencephalitis, if at all?
10. How is this disease related to the congenital rubella syndrome, if at all?
11. Name two other agents in the taxonomic group of the pathogen in this case.
12. Describe the pathogenesis of these other two agents.

Student Questions

Case 6 TB or Not TB

Rob W. was in his third year, his first clinical year in medicine. He had surgery as his first 8-week block and just now finished the medicine service. After his 8 weeks on medicine, he looked forward to a free block. The clinical years were more demanding than he thought. The long hours, the hurried hospital cafeteria meals, and none too tasty at that, had worn him down.

The free block didn't do much to improve his strength. He still felt tired, hadn't regained any of his lost weight, had actually lost a little more, and had a light cough.

Rob arranged a lung x-ray, which showed only a few calcified lesions, nothing more than you would expect from a lifelong resident of Memphis. Rob discussed this situation with the resident he'd had on his medical service, who recommended a skin test for tuberculosis. Rob said he had been PPD-negative when tested in the immunology laboratory last year.

Questions

1. What is a common cause of calcified lesions in the lung of a lifelong resident of Memphis?
2. Describe PPD. How does it differ from OT?
3. Describe the use of PPD and the interpretation of reactions to PPD.
4. Do calcified lesions eliminate tuberculosis and histoplasmosis from the differential diagnosis?
5. Why weren't skin tests for fungal infections requested?
6. What features of this case, if any, suggest mycoplasmal pneumonia?
7. How is the microbiologic diagnosis of tuberculosis established?
8. How is the microbiologic diagnosis of histoplasmosis established?

Student Questions

Case 7 Another College Complaint

Pre-finals anxiety was already widespread among the freshman class at Pax College. It had started right after the Thanksgiving vacation with lots of students complaining of headaches, sore throat, colds, and a miscellaneous collection of ills, including diarrhea.

Gwen was convinced she had something else. Her throat had been sore for several days. She felt tired and feverish and had swollen, tender lymph nodes "under the back of her chin." Gwen decided to visit the student health clinic.

The nurse recorded her vital signs as follows:

Temperature	100.8°F
Pulse	68
Respirations	19
Blood pressure	124/78 mm Hg

The student health physician confirmed the swollen submandibular lymph nodes and an inflamed pharynx coated with a slight gray-green exudate. He also noted a splenomegaly, but other physical findings were unremarkable.

Hematologic studies were performed with the following results:

Hematocrit	43%
Hemoglobin	15.4 g/dl
Red cells	5,100,000/mm^3
White cells	13,700/mm^3
Lymphocytes	58%
Monocytes	3%
Eosinophils	4%
Basophils	1%
Neutrophils	24%
Band cells	2%
Atypical lymphocytes	8%

The doctor ordered serologic tests and took a swab for throat cultures. He decided against liver function tests and told Gwen to return to her dorm, to rest, and to call back for the report of the serologic and bacteriologic tests the next day. When her diagnosis was confirmed, Gwen was advised that there was no specific treatment, that her recovery could be prolonged, and that, if needed, she could get medical authorization to withdraw from school and receive incomplete grades.

Questions

1. Is fatigue a prerequisite for contracting this illness?
2. What value toward the diagnosis are the physical findings?
3. What key clues are present in the laboratory findings?

4. Would you expect to recover beta-hemolytic streptococci from the throat cultures?
5. Describe the serologic tests you would request for this student.
6. Explain the nature of the antigens used in this test and their specificity in relationship to the etiologic agent.
7. Is recovery from this illness as prolonged as Gwen's physician suggests? Why?
8. What other conditions are associated with infections by this agent?
9. Gwen's physician prescribed only rest, yet other conditions associated with this agent are treatable with chemotherapeutics. Explain.
10. How does the pathogen in this illness enter the cells in which it resides?

Student Questions

Case 8 A Real Hep Professor

William W., a 43-year-old professor in the Economics Department, had spent the last 2 weeks in Thailand as a guest of the Royal Kha-Song University. His seminar series had gone well, and his guests had been very generous in providing first-class hotel accommodations. However, William prized his ability to locate restaurants off the beaten track that served "real" Thai food.

Two weeks after his return to the States, William noted that his urine was much darker than normal. He actually felt quite well, although it had taken several days to recover from his jet lag, and he felt a little more tired than normal. This dark urine frightened him, so he made an appointment with his doctor for the next day.

William denied using intravenous drugs or excessive use of alcohol. He also denied homosexual contacts. He had no recent contact with domestic or farm animals. He described his recent trip to Thailand, which prompted several questions from his doctor. A physical examination produced no significant information with the exception of a possible slight conjunctival icterus.

Urinalysis confirmed the brown color that William had described. The urine was clear and free of casts and cells. No protein or sugar was detected in the urine.

Blood was collected for biochemical and serologic tests. The results of the biochemical tests revealed enzyme elevations of alkaline phosphatase, aminotransferases, and bilirubin. From these data, William's diagnosis was quite certain and was later confirmed by the serologic tests.

Questions

1. What infectious diseases do you associate with a dark urine?
2. Which of these do you associate with the Orient?
3. Is this association with the Orient exclusive, or do these diseases appear elsewhere?
4. Could this be a zoonotic disease even though William had no recent contact with animals?
5. What serologic tests would be applied to assist in the diagnosis of this illness?
6. Are chemotherapeutics available to speed recovery from this disease?
7. What sequelae, if any, are associated with this illness?
8. Compare hepatitis virus A and hepatitis virus B transmission and disease.
9. Discuss the antibody response to hepatitis B virus.
10. What is non-A, non-B hepatitis?

Student Questions

Case 9 A Case of Pneumonia

Grant A., a 46-year-old accountant with leukemia, has been under treatment with cytotoxic drugs for 6 months. About 2 months after entering treatment, he developed herpes zoster. His therapy was reduced at that time, but later he had a case of thrush, which was successfully treated.

At the present time, Grant entered the hospital for a fever and dry cough that had developed over a period of several days. His current physical signs were as follows:

Temperature	102.2°F
Pulse	84
Respirations	24
Blood pressure	138/78 mm Hg

He appeared anemic, which was later confirmed by red cell count and hematocrit. His white cell count was low but with a normal differential. The physical examination noted breath sounds and rales in both lung fields. X-rays confirmed an infiltrate in both lower lung fields.

Cultures of blood and urine were unrevealing. Failure to raise a sputum prevented culture. Grant was started on erythromycin, but no improvement could be noted over the following 3 days.

Questions

1. What agents of pneumonia are more prevalent in adults?
2. What is herpes zoster infection?
3. Is cytotoxic therapy related to herpes zoster or the pneumonia?
4. Erythromycin is often used to treat legionellosis. Is this logical here?
5. Aren't blood cultures usually positive in cases of pneumonia?
6. Which pneumonias are associated with a dry cough and little sputum?
7. What is the relationship of thrush to this case?
8. After no improvement following 3 days of erythromycin, what would you do? Reculture? Change therapy?
9. Which pneumonias are associated with cytotoxic drug therapy?
10. Which animal parasites cause pneumonia?

Student Questions

Case 10 On the Track of Tracheitis

Only 2 days earlier Kevin had been the ideal baby boy. Though only $1^1/2$ years old, he was running not walking, jabbered almost constantly trying out newfound words, and eating every food he was offered.

But last night he began to cough, acted lethargic, and had a fever. This morning the pediatrician prescribed amoxicillin by telephone. This evening Kevin had a fever of 40°C, was having trouble breathing, and when seen in the emergency department was cyanotic and had developed stridor. Chest x-rays revealed a significant subglottal narrowing and infiltrates in both left lung lobes.

Kevin was taken to the operating room for a tracheoscopy. Heavy viscous and purulent secretions from the trachea were cultured. Parainfluenza 1 virus and *Staphylococcus aureus* were later isolated from the tracheal secretions. Blood cultures were negative. The hematology laboratory reported 9400 cells/mm^3 as the white blood cell count, of which 97% were neutrophils.

Questions

1. The dual viral and bacterial isolation suggests a symbiotic disease. Explain.
2. How do you isolate influenza and parainfluenza viruses?
3. How do you type the influenza viruses?
4. Discuss the hemagglutinin(s) and neuraminidase(s) of the influenza viruses.
5. Wasn't the treatment of Kevin a little overly dramatic? Explain.
6. Why wasn't this treated like an ordinary staphylococcal infection?
7. Is it possible to treat influenza virus infections?
8. Describe antigenic shift and drift among the influenza viruses.
9. What is the split flu vaccine?
10. Discuss typing of the parainfluenza viruses.

Student Questions

Case 11 Sleepless Nights

Amy, a 6-year-old, hadn't slept well the last two nights. On Thursday night, she woke up crying at 10:30 just when her parents were going to bed. Last night she woke up about 3 AM, crying and claiming her bottom itched. Her mother washed Amy's anal area and coated it with hand cream.

Saturday morning the family's physician was contacted. He telephoned a prescription to the local pharmacy for a mebendazole generic compound.

Questions

1. What is the estimated incidence of enterobiasis in the United States?
2. What is the life cycle of *Enterobius vermicularis*?
3. What is meant by the term *autoinfection*?
4. How does autoinfection occur in pinworm infections? In other helminth infections?
5. Is pinworm always a mild condition of anal pruritus?
6. How is pinworm customarily diagnosed?
7. What is mebendazole's mode of action?
8. What drugs are prescribed for helminth infections?
9. Compare nematodes and cestodes.
10. What helminth infections are common in the United States?

Student Questions

Case 12 Eye Can't See

Melissa, a 16-year-old high school girl, had been using daily-wear soft contact lenses for only 2 months. At first these seemed to be compatible with the goggles she wore when competing as a member of her high school swim team. After the swim meet Saturday, she noted a little more irritation in her right eye than could be accounted for by the chlorine-thick air of the natatorium. On Monday, her eye was much worse, and the swim team coach got her an appointment with the team physician.

The physician recommended topical corticosteroid treatment and therapy for a presumed herpes simplex keratitis. During the succeeding 4 weeks, Melissa gradually lost vision in her right eye and when seen by an ophthalmologist had a distinctive stromal keratitis. Melissa was sent to the Mid-State Ophthalmology Clinic, where a potential diagnosis of *Acanthamoeba* keratitis was made.

Questions

1. Discuss the pathogenesis of herpes simplex keratitis and conjunctivitis.
2. How are herpes simplex infections treated?
3. What is the meaning of type 1 versus type 2 herpes infections?
4. What role do herpes viruses have in oncogenesis?
5. Distinguish between *Acanthamoeba, Endamoeba*, and *Entamoeba*.
6. What are the free-living amoebae?
7. Discuss the etiology of primary amoebic meningoencephalitis.
8. Compare the prognosis of amoebic keratitis and meningoencephalitis.
9. In general, what therapies are recommended for treatment of protozoan infections due to amoeba and ciliated protozoa?
10. What are the major reservoirs of *Acanthamoeba*?

Student Questions

Case 13 The Duck Hunter Who Ducked

Ray met the three others at the All Nite Diner, from which they drove to the lake. They took their position in the duck blind. Ray took the south end of the blind. The raw northern wind meant that the ducks would probably swing in from the south. Through the clouds, daylight was just breaking as Ray pushed his face into the reeds covering the blind in front of his lookout position. Some of the reeds scratched at his right upper lip and cheek. A little discomfort, but nothing to complain about.

By 11 AM, Ray was happy to give up the hunt. They hadn't killed their limit, but Ray's lip was pretty irritated from ducking his face in and out of the reeds every time birds were in sight. His lips were chapped from the cold wind, and he was ready to head in.

During the evening of the next day, Ray noticed a little tingling feeling in his lips—just the area he irritated while hunting. The next morning three separate vesicles about 2 or 3 mm in diameter dotted that same area. The itching began, and Ray knew it would be a week or so before the crusty lesion dried up and was shed.

Questions

1. Did Ray acquire this infection while hunting? Where did he acquire it?
2. If not recently acquired, explain the condition of latency of this infection. Is latency curable?
3. Compare the herpes viruses that cause human infections.
4. Describe Burkitt's lymphoma in detail.
5. Other than Burkitt's lymphoma, what cancers are associated with herpes virus?
6. What other DNA viruses are potentially oncogenic?
7. What RNA viruses are potentially oncogenic?
8. How does herpes zoster relate to Ray's case?
9. Are all herpes infections treated with acyclovir?
10. Explain why high antibody titers fail to protect against herpes infections.

Student Questions

Review Questions

1. Which of the following parasites would be most likely encountered in a private clinical practice?

   A. *Ascaris lumbricoides*
   B. *Enterobius vermicularis*
   C. *Schistosoma mansoni*
   D. *Entamoeba histolytica*
   E. *Necator americanus*

2. Nosocomial infections may affect which hospitalized patients?

   A. Basically healthy patients having elective surgery
   B. Immunocompromised patients
   C. Newborn infants
   D. Patients treated with antibiotics
   E. All of the above

3. The etiologic agent of candidiasis is
   A. Rarely endogenous to the host
   B. Opportunistic
   C. Composed of septate hyphae in its mycelial phase
   D. Sensitive to chloramphenicol
   E. All of the above

4. A patient with a long-standing condition of cystic fibrosis yielded a gram-negative, blue-green pigmenting bacillus from cultures of sputum. This organism is most likely to be
   A. *Proteus vulgaris*
   B. *Pseudomonas aeruginosa*
   C. *Escherichia coli*
   D. An alpha-hemolytic *Haemophilus influenzae*
   E. *Bordetella pertussis*

5. The staphylococcal disease known as "toxic shock syndrome" is an example of
   A. A toxemia due to ingestion of preformed toxin
   B. A toxemia due to the production of a toxin by colonizing or infecting bacteria
   C. A local infection
   D. A septicemia
   E. A metastatic infection

6. Hepatitis B virus
   A. Infection is acquired from contaminated food or water
   B. Vaccines are highly protective
   C. Is also known as the delta agent
   D. Antigen in the blood is an indication the person will become a carrier
   E. Antibody in the blood is an indication the person is a carrier

7. Antibiotic-associated colitis is
   A. Also known as pseudomembranous, clindamycin-induced colitis
   B. Produced by *Clostridium difficile* cytotoxins
   C. Actually best treated by antibiotic therapy
   D. Characterized by bloody diarrhea, fever, and severe abdominal pain
   E. All of the above

8. Which one of the following is most likely to be isolated from blood when it is the etiologic agent of disease?
   A. *Vibrio cholerae*
   B. *Pseudomonas aeruginosa*
   C. *Escherichia coli*
   D. *Salmonella typhi*
   E. *Shigella sonnei*

9. Poliomyelitis virus

A. Has infectious RNA
B. Is inactivated in the Sabin type vaccine
C. In the Sabin vaccine cannot revert to the wild type
D. Answers A, B, and C are correct.
E. Answers A and C only are correct.

10. The Dane particle

A. Is the capsid of hepatitis A virus
B. Is the entire virion of hepatitis A virus
C. Is related to the Australia antigen
D. Was discovered in Denmark to be the cause of serum hepatitis
E. Is a common structure of types A, B, and non-A, non-B hepatitis viruses

II

Medical Immunology

11 Immunity

Immunity is generally considered as either a natural or innate condition, known variously also as inherited immunity or resistance, and includes acquired immunity, which is an adaptive response to infectious agents. Although this comparison is useful, it is equally useful to describe immunity as either antigen specific or nonspecific.

In the case of antigen-nonspecific immunity, two separate categories are discernable. The first comprises constitutive activities and permanent structures that would place antigen-nonspecific immunity with natural immunity in the traditional classification scheme. The skin as a mechanical barrier, acids in our sebaceous gland secretions, lysozyme in our tears and other body fluids, and the mucus and ciliated cells of our respiratory system would all be included here. These activities are not changed significantly in quantity nor does their mechanism of action become altered in response to differences in the antigenicity of the pathogens we encounter.

The second category of constitutive, antigen-nonspecific immunity includes the macrophages and neutrophils, both phagocytic cells, and the natural killer (NK) cells. These cells have a fixed pattern of behavior that follows their encounter with infectious agents regardless of the antigenic characteristics of the invader. Unlike the fixed nature of the cornified outer layers of our skin, or the locked behavior of ciliated cells of our respiratory system, the behavior of phagocytes and NK cells is modified by their contact with infectious agents. This change is unrelated to the antigenic nature of the pathogen and is still classified as antigen-nonspecific immunity. The ability of the antigen-specific B and T lymphocytes to influence both phagocytes and NK cells reveals that the latter can be indirectly influenced by an antigen-specific response, however.

Acquired immunity is an antigen-specific response that through the expression of inducible activities may influence components of natural immunity. The antigen-specific operators of acquired immunity are the T and B lymphocytes. The T cells exist in several subsets, among which the $CD4^+$ helper T (T_{H1}) cells may be considered the most essential because they influence the activity of the other T cell subsets—the cytotoxic CD8+ T lymphocytes (CTL or T_C), the suppressor T cells (T_S), and those T cells involved in delayed-type hypersensitivity (T_{DTH} or $CD4^+$ T_{H2} cells)—and the B and NK lymphocytes as well. The response of T cells to infectious agents is collected under the term *cell-mediated immunity*. This is separate from cell-mediated immunity as contributed by the phagocytes and NK cells.

The T_H cells also stimulate the response of B lymphocytes to antigen, a response that is characterized by the synthesis of immunoglobulins (antibodies). Since antigen-specific immunoglobulins are detected easily in the blood, this aspect of immunity is known as humoral immunity. Humoral immunity is customarily described as self-generated (active immunity) or contributed (passive immunity) to the individual in question.

The separation of humoral immunity into that which is self-acquired, the so-called active form of immunity, or that which is passively acquired permits an even further subdivision of immunity (Table 11-1). Naturally and artificially acquired active immunity depend on recovery from disease and immunity accomplished by immunization, respectively. Immunity acquired from another immune individual (passive immunity) can also be naturally (from maternal immunoglobulins) or artificially (from injections of immunoglobulins) acquired.

Active immunization has led to the elimination of smallpox and to a significant reduction in the incidence of many diseases such as yellow fever, whooping cough, poliomyelitis, and others. When the symptoms of an illness are due largely to exotoxins produced by the pathogen, toxoids in vaccines induce the synthesis of antitoxin (antibody to toxin). Toxoids have been very effective in preventing diphtheria and tetanus. Purified structural components of some microbes, such as the capsular polysaccharides of the pneumococcus, are often key antigens, in this instance as a vaccine against lobar pneumonia. The live but attenuated BCG (Bacille Calmette-Guérin) vaccine has had varied success in trials to reduce tuberculosis, probably due to failures to prepare and maintain the vaccine properly in the least successful trials.

Attenuated viral vaccines against mumps, measles, rubella, and poliomyelitis are used routinely to immunize U.S. citizens (Table 11-2), and an inactive form of the poliomyelitis vaccine is also used. The influenza and hepatitis B vaccines are recommended for special risk groups, the latter now being available as a recombinant vaccine.

Passive prophylactic immunization has proved successful in preventing hemolytic disease of the newborn and hepatitis A infections, but antisera used in other circumstances, such as for treatment of rabies, tetanus, or gas gangrene, have varied in their efficacy.

Other forms of immunity include adoptive immunization in which T and/or B cells or their precursors are transplanted into immunodeficient persons. An additional

Table 11-1. Classification of humoral immunity

Type of immunity	Means of acquisition
ACTIVE IMMUNITY	
Naturally acquired	Clinical or subclinical disease
Artificially acquired	Attenuated vaccine
	Inactivated or killed vaccine
	Toxoid or other purified antigen
PASSIVE IMMUNITY	
Naturally acquired	Transplacental IgG
Artificially acquired	Hyperimmune human or animal globulin

Table 11-2. Recommended immunizations for U.S. citizens*

Bacterial disease		Viral disease	
Pertussis	in DPT vaccine	Measles	in MMR vaccine
Diphtheria	in DPT vaccine	Mumps	in MMR vaccine
Tetanus	in DPT vaccine	Rubella	in MMR vaccine
Pneumonia		Poliomyelitis—Sabin or Salk	
		Influenza	
		Hepatitis B	

*Vaccines against bacterial meningitis, rabies, and tuberculosis are advised for special risk groups.

as yet unnamed method of acquiring immunity is through injections of colony-stimulating factors, interferons, and interleukins that activate inert cells of the recipient.

It should be added here that microbes have developed various methods to escape their host's immune response, including an intracellular lifestyle, steady modification of their surface antigens, shedding of soluble antigens that block host contact with that same antigen on the host, or secreting false receptors for interleukins.

Key Words and Phrases

Mastery of these words, phrases, and abbreviations used in discussion of immunity will be helpful when you consider problem cases in the later chapters.

Acquired immunity
Active immunity
Adoptive immunity
Anamnestic response
Antigenic drift
Antigenic shift
Anti-idiotypic vaccine
Antitoxin
Attenuated vaccine
Cell-mediated immunity
Chemotaxin
Colony-stimulating factor
Conjugated vaccine
Defensin
Hib vaccine
Humoral immunity
Hypochlorite ion
Immune adherence
Innate immunity
Interferon
Interleukin
Lymphotoxin
Lysozyme
Natural immunity
Natural killer cell
Nitric oxide
Opsonin
Oxidative burst
Passive immunity
Perforin
Phagocytosis
Polyvalent vaccine
Recombinant vaccine
Sabin vaccine

Salk vaccine
Split vaccine
Superantigen
Synthetic vaccine
T cell–dependent antigen
T cell–independent antigen
Toxoid

Abbreviations

ADCC
BCG
CTL
DPT
ELAM-1
ICAM-1
IFN-α
IL-1
MMR
NK cell
PRP
TNF-α

Information Sources

Books

Ades, E.W., and Lopez, C., editors: Natural killer cells and host defense, S. Karger Publishers, Inc., 1989, Farmington, CT.

Arnon, R., editor: Synthetic vaccines, CRC Press, Inc., 1987, Boca Raton.

Bos, J.D., editor: Skin immune system, CRC Press, Inc., 1990, Boca Raton.

Burd, R., Cody, C.S., and Dunn, D.L., editors: Immunotherapy of gram-negative bacterial sepsis, CRC Press, Inc., 1992, Boca Raton.

Chaouat, G., editor: Immunology of pregnancy, CRC Press, Inc., 1992, Boca Raton.

Cochrane, C.C., and Gimbrone, M.A., Jr., Cellular and molecular mechanisms of inflammation, Academic Press, Inc., 1990, San Diego.

Cruse, J.M., and Lewis, R.E., Jr., editors: Conjugate vaccines, S. Karger AG, 1989, Basel.

Cryz, S.J., editor: Vaccines and immunotherapy, Pergamon Press, 1991, Riverside, NJ.

Ellis, R.W., editor: Hepatitis B vaccines in clinical practice, Marcel Dekker, Inc., 1992, New York.

Kurstak, E., editor: Control of virus diseases, Marcel Dekker, Inc., 1992, New York.

Germanier, R., editor: Bacterial vaccines, Academic Press, Inc., 1984, Orlando.

Mizrabi, A., editor: Bacterial vaccines, Wiley-Liss, Inc., 1990, New York.

Mizrabi, A., editor: Viral vaccines, Wiley-Liss, Inc., 1990, New York.

Nelson, D.S.: Natural immunity, Academic Press, Inc., 1989, San Diego.

Plotkin, S.A., and Mortimer, E.A., Jr., editors: Vaccines, W.B. Saunders Publisher, 1988, Philadelphia.

Reynolds, C.W., and Wiltrout, R.H., editors: Functions of the natural immune system, Plenum Publishing Co., 1989, New York.

VanFurth, R., editor: Mononuclear phagocytes: characteristics, physiology and function, Martinum Nijhoff, 1985, Amsterdam.

Woodrow, G.C., and Levine, M.M., editors: New generation vaccines, Marcel Dekker, Inc., 1990, New York.

Zuckerman, A.J., editor: Recent developments in prophylactic immunizations, Kluwer Academic Publishers, 1989, Hingham, MA.

Reviews

Amstey, M.S.: The potential for maternal immunization to protect against neonatal infections, Semin. Perinatal. **15**:206, 1991.

Arnon, R., and Horwitz, R.J.: Synthetic peptides as vaccines, Curr. Opin. Immunol. **4**:449, 1992.

Atkinson, W.L., Orenstein, W.A., and Krugman, S.: The resurgence of measles in the United States, 1989–1990, Annu. Rev. Med. **43**:451, 1992.

Brown, F.: Vaccines, Curr. Opin. Immunol. **2**:392, 1990.

Dwyer, J.M.: Manipulating the immune system with immune globulin, N. Engl. J. Med. **326**:107, 1992.

Gordon, S., et al.: Macrophages in tissues and in vitro, Curr. Opin. Immunol. **4**:25, 1992.

Graw, G.E., and Modlin, R.L.: Immune mechanisms in bacterial and parasitic diseases: protective immunity versus pathology, Curr. Opin. Immunol. **3**:480, 1991.

Hill, D.R.: Immunizations, Infect. Dis. Clin. North Am., **6**:291, 1992.

Lanier, L.L., and Phillips, J.H.: Natural killer cells, Curr. Opin. Immunol. **4**:38, 1992.

McGee, J.R., et al.: The mucosal immune system from fundamental concepts to vaccine development, Vaccine **10**:75, 1992.

Melick, D.R.: Synthetic peptides: prospects for vaccine development, Semin. Immunol. **2**:307, 1990.

Sher, A., and Coffman, R.L.: Regulation of immunity to parasites by T cells and T cell–derived cytokines, Annu. Rev. Immunol. **10**:385, 1992.

Young, D.B.: Heat shock proteins: immunity and autoimmunity, Curr. Opin. Immunol. **4**:396, 1992.

Zurbriggen, A., and Fujinami, R.S.: Immunity to viruses, Curr. Opin. Immunol. **2**:347, 1990.

Case 1 Officer Briggs's Dilemma

Mr. H. Briggs, health officer of a community of 65,000 inhabitants, was concerned about the risk of hepatitis B infection in city employees who worked in the sewer management or sewage treatment divisions of the city government. He decided to arrange for the immunization of 37 employees in these divisions before expanding this benefit to employees in the police, fire, and city health departments. A private firm was contracted to give three 0.1-ml doses of recombinant hepatitis B vaccine to all 37 employees. The vaccine was to be given by the intradermal rather than the intramuscular route. The firm would determine if seroconversion followed the vaccination and would give one more dose of vaccine to nonresponders. Unfortunately only 7 of the vaccinees converted, and Health Officer Briggs wondered if this new vaccine was really any good.

Questions

1. What are the source and nature of the recombinant hepatitis B vaccines?
2. Is the recombinant vaccine highly effective?
3. How were previous hepatitis B vaccines prepared?
4. What health risks were possible with the older vaccines? Were any of these risks realized?
5. What antigens of the hepatitis B virus are useful in determining whether immunity exists?
6. What antigens are useful in evaluating acute, chronic, and carrier status of hepatitis B infections?
7. What serologic tests are used to evaluate immunity to hepatitis B virus infections?
8. What potential benefit other than protection against hepatitis may be derived from active immunization?
9. What is the status of passive immunization against B-type hepatitis?
10. The intradermal route of immunization is often considered a suitable route. Can you suggest why it was unsuccessful in this instance?
11. What is the status of immunization against other forms of viral hepatitis?

Student Questions

Case 2 Polio in the Americas

Dr. Carillo, in charge of the Mexican effort of the Pan American Health Organization (PAHO) plan to eradicate poliomyelitis in the Americas, was pleased with the results his assistants had prepared for him. Since 1985, when the incidence of polio in Mexico was 0.07 cases/100,000 persons, it was now reduced, through the use of the oral polio vaccine, to a figure so low it had no statistical meaning. Now at midyear of 1990, there had been only one proven case of wild polio in Mexico.

Dr. Carillo was scheduled to give a talk to members of the Mexican-American Institute tomorrow. He wondered if he should discuss the risks of the oral polio vaccine and why it was often preferred to the inactive or killed vaccine.

Questions

1. Discuss the nature and content of the oral poliomyelitis vaccine.
2. Discuss the nature and content of the inactivated (killed) poliomyelitis vaccine.
3. How can one be immune to polio and still serve as a source of this disease?
4. What is the difference between poliovirus infection and disease? What is the meaning of the term "wild polio"?
5. How does vaccine-associated paralytic polio occur?
6. Contrast mucosal and humoral antibody immunity.
7. What are the recommendations relative to booster immunizations against poliomyelitis?
8. Can the polio vaccines be given as combined vaccines against other diseases?
9. The poliovirus is an enterovirus. Are vaccines available against other enteroviruses?
10. For what viral diseases are attenuated vaccines available?

Student Questions

Case 3 Flu Epidemic

The fax was received at the Centers for Disease Control communications center at 10 AM local time. It was hand-carried to the respiratory disease section and passed on to Dr. Rodney Pattner's secretary in the virology unit, who stamped it received at 10:20 AM. She paged Dr. Pattner in the level 3 biosafety laboratory, and 20 minutes later he was reading the fax. As he put the paper down, he asked his secretary to call a special staff meeting of the influenza group for 1 PM.

As the group began to assemble in the conference room, the main rumor that emerged was that a new flu strain had cropped up somewhere. Dr. Pattner soon confirmed this. A highly virulent influenza A H2N2 strain had been identified at the influenza monitoring station in Copenhagen. Already 12 people had died, and at least 279 others were ill of symptoms harmonious with those of viral influenza. Pattner explained that last winter's vaccine would be useless against the new strain, and although it was now October 1, new split vaccine could be available in a month.

Questions

1. What is the role of influenza viruses A, B, and C in human disease?
2. What is the meaning of H2N2?
3. How are newly isolated strains of influenza virus designated?
4. What is meant by antigenic drift and antigenic shift?
5. What is the split influenza virus vaccine, and what are its advantages?
6. How is it possible to have flu vaccines available in such a short time when this is not possible for most viral diseases?
7. Why is immunity to pathogens of mucosal surfaces, in general, considered to be poor?
8. Which viral diseases are combatted with killed (inactive) vaccines?

Student Questions

Case 4 Pneumo Vaccine

The Clarion County Rest Home had 47 residents, only 4 of whom were less than 65 years of age. Twelve of the 18 male residents were cigarette smokers. Of the 47 residents, 6 had chronic respiratory problems—3 asthmatics and 3 with past lung resection. Two of the residents had diabetes. Two had rheumatoid arthritis, for which they received steroid therapy.

Head Nurse Wendelling called the county health officer with this information in preparation for his visit and administration of the pneumococcal vaccine.

Questions

1. What is the nature of the current pneumococcal vaccine?
2. What is the recommendation for the use of this vaccine in the different persons mentioned above?
3. Are annual or other booster doses of the vaccine recommended? Why or why not?
4. What other patient groups should receive the pneumococcal vaccine?
5. What is the IgM and/or IgG response to this vaccine?
6. Is the pneumococcal vaccine a TI antigen or TD antigen?
7. What components of the cellular immune system contribute to antipneumococcal immunity?
8. Discuss phagocytosis as a component of pneumococcal immunity.
9. Describe the steps in the oxidative pathway used by phagocytes to kill bacteria.
10. What are opsonins?

Student Questions

Case 5 PAIDS

Female baby Nixon had PAIDS (pediatric acquired immune deficiency syndrome) as the result of a transplacental infection from her mother. As yet, the infant had shown no symptoms of the disease, but serologic tests had identified the presence of HIV type 1 virus in her blood.

This was the first PAIDS infant that Dr. Cooper had encountered, and he was uncertain how to handle the immunization program for this child.

Questions

1. What is the routine immunization schedule for normal, healthy infants and children?
2. Explain the background for omitting the smallpox vaccine from that list.
3. What is the immunization program for asymptomatic PAIDS patients?

4. Does the recommended vaccine listing change if the PAIDS patient is symptomatic?
5. Multidrug-resistant tuberculosis is a threat to immunosuppressed persons. Describe the vaccine against tuberculosis and its use in healthy subjects and those with symptomatic PAIDS or AIDS.
6. Are vaccines available or in development against *Pneumocystis* infection, toxoplasmosis, cryptococcosis, or other common diseases of AIDS patients?
7. What is the status of vaccine development against AIDS?
8. Does immunity to HIV-1 confer immunity against HIV-2?
9. What antigens in blood are consistent with a diagnosis of AIDS?
10. What antibodies in blood are consistent with a diagnosis of AIDS?

Student Questions

Review Questions

1. Which of the following diseases is combatted by the use of an attenuated, live vaccine?
   A. Tuberculosis
   B. Tetanus
   C. Pertussis
   D. Pneumococcal pneumonia
   E. Hepatitis B
2. An advantage of a recombinant vaccine over other vaccines is
   A. The ease by which they can be produced
   B. Their use as a vaccine against common bacteria or yeasts
   C. The ability to select a single important antigen for production by recombinant DNA technology
   D. That they can be more easily used with adjuvants
   E. That they stimulate both B and T cells

3. Which of the following is **not** considered a polyvalent vaccine?

A. Pneumococcal pneumonia vaccine
B. Salk poliomyelitis vaccine
C. Sabin poliomyelitis vaccine
D. Mumps vaccine
E. The DPT vaccine

4. Which of the following is **not** a part of innate (natural) immunity?

A. Lysozyme
B. Complement
C. Transplacental immunity bestowed on the fetus
D. Phagocytosis
E. Defensins

5. Defensin(s) is/are

A. A collection of antimicrobial peptides present in granulocytes
B. The major cytotoxic agent of NK cells
C. A part of the oxygen-dependent activity of phagocytes
D. An acute phase protein
E. Part of the external defense system

6. The vaccine against *Haemophilus influenzae* infections

A. That contains only PRP is suitable for infants less than 1 year of age
B. Known as the conjugate vaccine contains PRP plus either diphtheria toxoid or meningococcal protein
C. Also provides protection against pneumococcal pneumonia because of its polysaccharide content
D. Is used primarily to prevent the earliest bacterial cause of meningitis in young infants
E. Contains antigens from *H. influenzae* types A, B, and C

7. Circulating antigen-specific antibody is most protective against which of the following?

A. Respiratory diseases of viral etiology
B. Diarrheas of bacterial etiology
C. Diseases where LPS causes the most significant symptom
D. The systemic effects of exotoxins
E. Fungal diseases

8. Myeloperoxidase of neutrophils

A. Catalyzes the reaction of H_2O_2 and CI ions to form OCI^- and H_2O
B. Forms the only toxic oxygen product found in neutrophils
C. Acts on the superoxide anion
D. Forms the superoxide anion as a major enzyme end product
E. None of the above

9. Which of the following is an example of adoptive immunity?

A. Injection of hyperimmune gamma globulin to prevent hepatitis A
B. A booster injection of tetanus toxoid
C. Successful bone marrow grafting into an immunodeficient person
D. Transplacental passage of IgG
E. None of the above

10. A major protective mechanism used by NK cells in innate immunity is

A. Lysozyme
B. Antibody-dependent cellular cytotoxicity (ADCC)
C. Phagocytosis
D. Secretion of tumor necrosis factor alpha (TNF-α)
E. None of the above

12 Immunoassays

Serologic assays and cytologic assays represent the two major forms of immunoassay. Typically, serologic assays are used to identify or quantitate the amount of antibody in a patient's serum, though some tests are designed to detect or measure antigen present in urine, spinal fluid, or some other specimen from the patient. The cytologic tests are intended to enumerate or determine the functional status of B lymphocytes, T lymphocytes, or phagocytic cells.

Blood banks are the site of most serologic assays simply because blood group determinations are performed on most hospital patients and because blood to be used in transfusion is evaluated for several infectious agents in addition to hematologic determinations.

The availability of high-titered antibody preparations, some of which are monoclonal, has favored the development of nephelometric assays that are both rapid and highly sensitive (Table 12-1). These tests rely only on the combination of antibody with antigen, a feature that allows the results of the assay to be determined very quickly. Most other serologic tests must pass through a second, aggregative phase before they

Table 12-1. The relative sensitivity of serologic tests to detect antigen

Highly sensitive
Radioimmunoassay (RIA)
Enzyme-linked immunosorbent assay (ELISA)
Passive agglutination or hemagglutination
Passive agglutination or hemagglutination inhibition
Intermediate sensitivity
Agglutination
Hemagglutination
Nephelometry
Radial immunodiffusion
Lower sensitivity
Fluid precipitation
Immunoelectrophoresis
Ouchterlony immunodiffusion
Fluorescent antibody tests

can be interpreted, and this requires time. Radial immunodiffusion and immunoelectrophoretic assays are examples of precipitation tests in which both stages (combination and aggregation) are necessary to yield a positive test. The former is a useful quantitative method and the latter a much used qualitative procedure. Ouchterlony double diffusion assay, another type of precipitation test, is still used in special circumstances. Fluid precipitation tests are relatively insensitive and seldom used.

The era of radioimmunoassays (RIA) is giving way rapidly to various adaptations of ELISA (enzyme-linked immunosorbent assay) methods. For many experimental purposes, ELISA tests are often run in concavity trays, but various dot-blotting methods with or without electrophoretic separation of antigen mixtures, as in HIV identification, are now popular because of their rapidity, sensitivity, and simplicity. The enhanced sensitivity of ELISA-blotting is attributable to the use of avidin-biotin, protein A, or second antibody amplification where one of these is the enzyme-labeled reagent.

Fluorescent antibody methods, such as the fluorescent antinuclear antibody (FANA) tests, so useful in the study of autoimmune diseases, are also of use in the diagnosis of infectious diseases.

Agglutination tests, once so useful in measuring the immune response of patients to bacterial infections through the use of acute and convalescent serum samples, are not now extensively used. Passive agglutination tests with antigen-coated latex particles (e.g., tests for the presence of group A streptococci) are faster and no more expensive. Passive agglutination inhibition tests to determine pregnancy already have a long history of home use. Many variations of these pregnancy kits are latex agglutination procedures often labeled as immunochromatographic tests.

The area of cellular immunology is an area in which exceptional advancements have been made. No longer restricted to mere enumeration of lymphocytes, immunologists can distinguish these cells as B or T cells and identify important subtypes—$CD4^+$ or $CD8^+$ T cells, IgD^+ B cells, and so on. Advancements in both monoclonal antibody technology and flow cytometry have combined to enable this. Unfortunately the cost of the equipment necessary to conduct these assays denies their use in most clinical laboratories.

Key Words and Phrases

Acute serum sample
Agglutination
Antinuclear antibody
Avidin-biotin enhancement
Bacterial agglutination
Biotin-avidin (streptavidin)
Blot test
Capture assay
Competitive inhibition assay
Complement fixation
Convalescent serum sample
Counterimmunoelectrophoresis
Cross-reacting antigen
Crossed immunoelectrophoresis
Enzyme-linked immunosorbent assay
Flagellar antigen
Flow cytometry
Fluorescent antibody test

Forssman antigen
H antigen
Hapten inhibition test
Hemagglutination
Heterophile antigen
Immunoblot assay
Immunochromatography
Immunoelectrophoresis
Mancini test
Microcytotoxicity test
Mixed lymphocyte reaction
Nephelometry
Neutralization test
Nitroblue tetrazolium reductase
O antigen
Ouchterlony immunodiffusion
Passive agglutination
Passive agglutination inhibition
Postzone
Precipitation
Primary antibody
Protein A
Prozone
Quellung reaction
Radial immunodiffusion
Radioimmunoassay
Rocket immunoelectrophoresis
Rise in titer
Second antibody
Solid phase assay
Somatic antigen
Weil-Felix reaction
Western blot test
Widal test

Abbreviations

ELISA
FAB
FANA
IEP
NBT
RAST
RIA
RIST

Information Sources

Numerous recent books and review articles are available in the area of immunoassays and will be valuable in solving the problem cases in this chapter.

Books

Bjerrum, O.J., and Heegaard, N.H.H., editors: CRC handbook of immunoblotting of proteins, CRC Press, Inc., 1988, Boca Raton.

Bullock, G.R., and Petrusz, P., editors: Techniques in immunocytochemistry, Academic Press, Inc., 1989, San Diego.

Chard, T.: An introduction to radioimmunoassay and related techniques, Elsevier Science Publishers, 1990, Amsterdam.

Coligan, J.E., et al., editors: Current protocols in immunology, Greene Publishing Associates, 1991, New York.

Dunbar, B.S.: Two-dimensional electrophoresis and immunological techniques, Plenum Press, Inc., 1987, New York.

Goers, J.: Immunochemical techniques laboratory manual, Academic Press, Inc., 1992, San Diego.

Grange, J.M., Fox, A., and Morgan, N.L., editors: Immunological techniques in microbiology, Blackwell Scientific Publications, 1987, Oxford.

Grogan, W.M., and Collins, J.M.: Guide to flow cytometry, Marcel Dekker, 1990, New York.

Harbeck, R.J., and Giclas, P.C.: Diagnostic immunology laboratory manual, Raven Press, Inc., 1991, New York.

Larsson, L.-I., editor: Enzyme-immunoassay, CRC Press, Inc., 1980, Boca Raton.

Lefkovits, I., and Pernis, B., editors: Immunological methods, vol. 1–5, Academic Press, Inc., 1985, San Diego.

Lennette, E.H., editor: Laboratory diagnosis of viral infections, edition 2, Marcel Dekker, Inc., 1991, New York.

Phillips, T.M.: Analytical techniques in immunochemistry, Marcel Dekker, Inc., 1992, New York.

Polak, J.M., and Priestley, J.V., editors: Electron microscopic immunocytochemistry, Oxford University Press, 1992, Oxford.

Rose, N.R., et al., editors: Manual of clinical laboratory immunology, ASM, 1992, Washington.

Sternberger, L.A.: Immunocytochemistry, edition 3, John Wiley & Sons, 1988, New York.

Weir, D.M., et al., editors: Handbook of experimental immunology, edition 4, 4 volumes, Blackwell Scientific Publications, 1986, Oxford.

Yazdi, H.M.: Diagnostic immunocytochemistry and electron microscopy, Igaku-Shoin, 1992, New York.

Zola, H.: Laboratory methods in immunology, CRC Press, Inc., 1990, Boca Raton.

Reviews

Battye, F.L., and Shortman, K.: Flow cytometry and cell separation procedures, Curr. Opin. Immunol. **3**:238, 1991.

Diamandis, E.P., and Christopoulos, T.K.: The biotin–(Strept) avidin system: principles and applications in biotechnology, Clin. Chem. **37**:625, 1991.

Elkins, R.P., and Chu, F.W.: Multianalyte microspot immunoassay: microanalytical "compact disk" of the future, Clin. Chem. **37**:1955, 1991.

June, C.H.: Analysis of lymphocyte activation and metabolism by flow cytometry, Curr. Opin. Immunol. **4**:200, 1992.

Miller, J.J., and Valdes, R., Jr.: Approaches to minimizing interference by cross-reacting molecules in immunoassays, Clin. Chem. **37**:144, 1991.

Walker, M.R., Stott, R.A., and Thorpe, G.H.G.: Enzyme-labeled antibodies in bioassays, Methods Biochem. Anal. **36**:179, 1992.

Case 1 Born to Shop

Gretchen B. was 33 years old and still considered herself a newlywed. She and Mel had been married almost a year and a half. Because both of them were in their 30s when they married, they wanted to start their family after their first year of marriage. From the way breakfast went down and then came back up, Gretchen thought everything must be on schedule. Morning sickness had been a daily event this week. Gretchen finished dressing and took the car to Sav-Bucks Drugstore, where she pondered over which pregnancy kit to buy.

Questions

1. What is the antigen in the pregnancy home test kits?
2. Is the antigen or the antibody coated on the indicator particle, or is it bound to some other surface?
3. Is the test an agglutination test, passive agglutination, passive agglutination inhibition test, or ELISA test?
4. What is immunochromatography?
5. What other medical tests depend on passive agglutination?
6. What other medical tests depend on passive agglutination inhibition?
7. How does the sensitivity of passive agglutination or passive agglutination inhibition tests compare to other serologic procedures?
8. Which is most sensitive—RIA or ELISA tests?
9. How are tests to detect ovulation arranged in terms of the antigen, antigen carrier (if any), antiserum, and procedure?
10. What is the reliability of pregnancy home test kits?

Student Questions

Case 2 Not Wrist, But RAST

Jim F. returned from the laboratory animal quarters with red, watery eyes and a runny nose. His wrists and hands were itching and inflamed from handling the animals. For the past month he had been doing experiments with guinea pigs, checking on them nearly every day. Earlier this week he started sneezing as soon as he entered the animal quarters, but now he had a full-blown allergy.

During consultation with an allergist, Jim explained that he had been bothered by hay fever since early childhood but that about the time he entered college this didn't seem to bother him as much as in the past. The allergist suggested a large series of diagnostic skin tests or the alternative of RAST tests. Since Jim had a real phobia of needles, he chose the RAST test.

Questions

1. What is the RAST test?
2. How can the **quantity** of IgE for an allergen be determined by the RAST test?
3. How is anti-IgE prepared? Is pure IgE used as the antigen?
4. Is the RAST test usually performed as an RIA test? Why or why not?
5. Compare the RAST test to the RIST test.
6. What tests are used to determine the total amount of IgE in a serum?
7. Can these same tests be used to measure antigen-specific IgE?
8. What type of serologic reactions result from the combination of IgE with antigen?
9. Describe the passive skin test used to detect IgE in serum.
10. How can RAST, RIST, or skin tests be used successfully to monitor desensitization?

Student Questions

Case 3 Blue but Doing OK

Amy L. had suffered far too many bacterial infections than was typical for a 4-year-old. Although she had otitis media only once, she had been afflicted with several episodes of sore throat, sinusitis, and other upper respiratory infections. Her pediatrician had been concerned about this earlicr and had ordered a nitroblue tetrazolium (NBT) reductase test last year. The results of the NBT test were normal. Now he decided to order a complete immunoglobulin profile.

Questions

1. Is serum immunoelectrophoresis (IEP) adequate to determine a patient's immunoglobulin profile?
2. How is an IEP test on serum conducted?
3. What tests would be recommended to determine immunoglobulin concentrations?
4. Is the radial immunodiffusion test advisable here? How is this test conducted and interpreted?
5. What are the normal immunoglobulin levels for a 4-year-old child?
6. How do immunoglobulin levels change with age?
7. How would you explain elevated IgG and IgM levels in Amy's case?
8. Would you expect IgA to be elevated or decreased?
9. How do you explain Amy's apparent freedom from a heightened incidence of viral infections?
10. Describe the nitroblue tetrazolium reductase test.

Student Questions

Case 4 AIDS—Eastwood and Western Blot

Martin Eastwood, a 27-year-old purchaser for the Rangel Brothers department store chain, had been slowly losing weight for the past 4 months. As a homosexual who had practiced "safe sex" only in the past few months, he was fully aware of his probable diagnosis. After an examination at his physician's office, he was told that his physical symptoms of weight loss, malaise, and lymphadenopathy coupled with his sexual history strongly suggested a diagnosis of AIDS. His physician suggested that they draw a blood sample and go directly to the Western blot test and skip presumptive testing for HIV.

Questions

1. What is the immunologic basis of the latex agglutination test for AIDS? Is this a presumptive or a confirmed test?
2. Describe the ELISA test as it is used for the diagnosis of AIDS.
3. What enzymes are used in ELISA tests?
4. How is the biotin-avidin (streptavidin) system used to improve the sensitivity of ELISA tests?
5. Describe the source and use of protein A to enhance AIDS tests.
6. What HIV antigens are employed in Western blot tests?
7. Describe the procedure of Western blot tests.
8. What antibodies are typically found in early and late AIDS patients?
9. Why isn't a low T lymphocyte count considered a confirmed diagnostic test for AIDS?
10. How is flow cytometry used simultaneously to enumerate $CD4^+$ and $CD8^+$ lymphocytes?
11. Which antibodies to which antigens are considered diagnostic of AIDS?

Student Questions

Case 5 Keep on Truckin'

Manuel M. had not worked for the past 10 days because of a light fever, headache, and myalgia. Last night he had a high fever, chills, and diarrhea. This morning he noticed several pink spots, all less than $^1/_2$ inch in diameter, clustered on his abdomen. Because of the persistent fever and diarrhea, he consulted his physician.

The physician made a tentative diagnosis of typhoid fever on the basis of the symptoms and the knowledge that Manuel, a truck driver for the Tex-Mex Transport Lines, had just returned 2 weeks ago from an extended trip to Mexico and had eaten often from street vendors. Although both blood and stool cultures for *Salmonella typhi* would later prove negative, other laboratory data—leukocytosis and elevated serum transaminases—were in harmony with the diagnosis. A serum sample was collected. Manuel was placed on sulfamethoxazole-trimethoprim and asked to return for a second serum sample on Monday, 12 days hence.

Questions

1. What are the important antigens of *Salmonella typhi* in relation to its virulence and immune response?
2. What is the relationship of lipopolysaccharide (LPS) to these antigens?
3. Discuss LPS, including its rough and smooth forms, in relation to immunity against *Salmonella* infections.
4. What is the Widal test?
5. What is meant by the term *febrile agglutinins*?
6. Describe the physical form of agglutination tests in relation to the structure of flagellated bacteria.
7. Describe *Salmonella* mutants that have been tested as vaccines.
8. What routes of immunization best stimulate intestinal immunity?
9. Describe the structure and synthesis of secretory IgA.
10. What is the meaning of the term *rise in titer* from the acute to the convalescent serum sample?
11. How are agglutination tests used to identify unknown cultures of bacteria?

Student Questions

Review Questions

1. One advantage of indirect fluorescent antibody assays compared to direct tests is the following:

A. Fewer incubations are required in indirect tests.
B. Indirect tests are more sensitive.
C. Indirect tests use fewer reagents and are thus less expensive.
D. Both antigen and antibody are labeled in the indirect tests, thus making these tests more sensitive.
E. Indirect tests can be applied to immunodiffusion tests, whereas direct tests cannot.

2. The functional integrity of phagocytic cells can be assessed by all of the following **except**

A. Microbicidal assay
B. Nitroblue tetrazolium test
C. Chemotaxis assay
D. Rosette test
E. None of the above

3. Functional assessment of T lymphocytes includes

A. Erythrocyte rosette assay
B. Surface immunoglobulin assay
C. Concanavalin A mitogen response
D. Serum immunoglobulin determination
E. Enumeration of $CD8^+$ cells

4. The best method for assessing the total number of B lymphocytes is

A. Quantitative immunoglobulin levels
B. Fc receptor assay
C. Erythrocyte rosette assay
D. Surface immunoglobulin assay
E. Concanavalin A mitogen response

5. Which of the following antibody fragments will precipitate with antigen?

A. Fc
B. Fab
C. $F(ab')_2$
D. Fd
E. Fc′

6. Positive delayed-type skin hypersensitivity tests depend on

A. Active T cells and active monocytes (macrophages)
B. Active T cells only
C. Active B cells
D. Active T and active B cells
E. Active B cells and active monocytes (macrophages)

7. Passive agglutination inhibition tests require

A. Antigen attached to a particular carrier
B. Free antigen preincubated with antibody
C. A preliminary titration of the antibody with an antigen-carrier conjugate
D. Answers A and B only
E. Answers A, B, and C

8. The primary purpose of diluting an antiserum in serologic tests is to

A. Avoid an extensive prozone
B. Avoid an extensive postzone
C. Broaden the zone of optimal proportions
D. Establish the exact equivalence point easily
E. All of the above

9. Which of the following can be considered an electrophoretic variant of radial immunodiffusion?

A. Counterimmunoelectrophoresis
B. Western blot tests
C. Rocket immunoelectrophoresis
D. Crossed immunoelectrophoresis
E. Ouchterlony immunodiffusion assays

13 Immunodeficiency

A genetic inability to synthesize the required cellular components of the immune system or a failure of those cells to function normally increases the susceptibility of an individual to infectious disease. This is described as a primary immunodeficiency state. Likewise, an impairment of the immune defense network through exposure to radiation, cytotoxic drug treatment, or infection may also produce an immunodeficiency, in these cases defined as an acquired or secondary immunodeficiency.

Analysis of individuals deficient in one of the four major areas in which immunity is based—(1) B cell and immunoglobulin production, (2) T cell and immune regulation, (3) the phagocytic cell systems, and (4) the complement system—has revealed significant differences in the kind of infectious disease afflicting each group (Table 13-1). For example, an increase in intracellular-dwelling bacterial infections, viral infections, or fungal infections often indicates a deficit in the T cell component. A deficiency in T cells may also result in an increased incidence of bacterial infections, since immunoglobulin production by B cells is regulated by T cells and these antibodies are frequently the basis of immunity to bacterial infections. Complement and phagocytic cell deficiencies are most frequently associated with an increase in bacterial infections.

When a deficiency arises at the T cell level, a number of diagnostic aids can be used to define the extent of the disease. Among these are the enumeration of peripheral blood lymphocytes, the response of these cells to T cell mitogens, such as concanavalin A, and the ability of the patient to demonstrate prior sensitization or to become sensitized to agents that typically provoke a delayed-type hypersensitivity.

B cell deficiencies may be expressed by a lowered peripheral blood lymphocyte count, but specific enumeration of these cells is preferred. Fortunately, the presence of immunoglobulin in serum is easily done and reflects past B cell function. Current B cell function can be assayed by the current response to vaccines or mitogens.

Phagocytic cell function is evaluated by phagocytic assays or the nitroblue tetrazolium reductase test, which is an indirect measurement of the oxidative killing potential of these cells.

Titration of the hemolytic potential of a serum is used to establish its complement content. Individual components of the complement system can be quantitated serologically.

Of the four categories of immunodeficiency, only the pure B cell deficiency states are easily corrected with pooled gamma globulin. Some phagocytic conditions have

Table 13-1. Major immunodeficiency states

B cell and immunoglobulin deficiency, reflected by an increase in extracellular bacterial infections
Transient neonatal hypogammaglobulinemia
Bruton's X-linked agammaglobulinemia
Common variable hypogammaglobulinemia
Immunoglobulin A deficiency
T cell deficiencies, reflected by an increase in many viral, fungal, and intracellular bacterial infections
Nezelof syndrome
DiGeorge syndrome
Wiskott-Aldrich syndrome
Ataxia-telangiectasia
Purine enzyme deficiency (adenosine deaminase and purine nucleotide phosphorylase)
AIDS
Phagocytic deficiency, reflected by an increase in bacterial diseases
Chronic granulomatous disease
Chédiak-Higashi syndrome
Myeloperoxidase deficiency
Leukocyte adhesion deficiency
Lazy leukocyte syndromes
Glucose-6-phosphate dehydrogenase deficiency
Complement and complement regulatory deficiencies, reflected by an increase in bacterial infections
Hereditary angioneurotic edema
Paroxysmal nocturnal hemoglobinuria
Late-acting component deficiency

responded to therapy with colony-stimulating factors, but this is still somewhat experimental. Complement deficiencies are not treated, but deficiency of C1 INH of the complement system is correctable with danazol.

Although bone marrow or thymus grafting has successfully repaired some T cell deficiency conditions, this always has the risk of graft-versus-host reactions or unexpected transmission of latent infections. Adenosine deaminase deficiency is treatable with special forms of the enzyme. AIDS is treatable with drugs but cannot be cured. Chronic mucocutaneous candidiasis responds to treatment with lymphocyte extracts. T cell deficiencies are the most difficult of the deficiency conditions to repair.

Key Words and Phrases

On completion of this chapter, you should be able to explain the meaning of all the following terms.

Actin deficiency
Adenosine deaminase
Ataxia-telangiectasia
Bare lymphocyte syndrome
Bruton's disease
C1 INH inhibitor
Chédiak-Higashi syndrome
Chronic granulomatous disease
Chronic mucocutaneous candidiasis
Colony-stimulating factors
Common variable hypogammaglobulinemia
Cytochrome b_{558}
Decay accelerating factor
DiGeorge syndrome
Glucose-6-phosphate dehydrogenase deficiency
Hereditary angioneurotic edema
Hyperimmunoglobulinemia E
Job's syndrome
Late-acting complement component
Lazy leukocyte syndrome
Leukocyte adhesion deficiency
Myeloperoxidase
NADPH oxidase
Neonatal hypogammaglobulinemia
Nezelof syndrome
Nitroblue tetrazolium reductase test
Paroxysmal nocturnal hemoglobinuria
Purine enzyme deficiency
Purine nucleotide phosphorylase
Selective hypogammaglobulinemia
Severe combined immunodeficiency
Superoxide dismutase
Transfer factor
Tuftsin deficiency
Wiskott-Aldrich syndrome
X-linked hypogammaglobulinemia

Abbreviations

ADA
AIDS
C1 INH
CGD
ELAM-1
IL-1
LAD
NBT
PNP
SCID
TNF-α

Information Sources

Books

Gupta, S., and Griscelli, C., editors: New concepts in immunodeficiency diseases, John Wiley & Sons, 1993, Chichester.

Samter, M., et al., editors: Immunologic diseases, edition 4, Little, Brown and Co., 1988, Boston.

Stiehm, E.R., editor: Immunologic disorders in infants and children, edition 3, W.B. Saunders Co., 1989, Philadelphia.

Webster, A.D.B.: Immunodeficiency and disease, Kluwer Academic Publishers, 1988, Dordrecht.

Wedgwood, R.J., Rosen, F.S., and Paul, N.W., editors: Primary immunodeficiency disease, Alan R. Liss, 1983, New York.

Reviews

Anderson, D.C., and Springer, T.A.: Leukocyte adhesion deficiency: an inherited defect in the Mac-1, LFA-1, and p150, 95 glycoproteins, Annu. Rev. Med. **38**:175, 1987.

Colten, H.R., and Rosen, F.S.: Complement deficiencies, Annu. Rev. Immunol. **10**:809, 1992.

Conley, M.E.: Molecular approaches to analysis of X-linked immunodeficiencies, Annu. Rev. Immunol. **10**:215, 1992.

de Saint Basile, G., and Fisher, A.: X-linked immunodeficiencies: clues to genes involved in T- and B-cell differentiation, Immunol. Today **12**:456, 1991.

Dinauer, M.C., and Orkin, S.H.: Chronic granulomatous disease, Annu. Rev. Med. **43**:117, 1992.

Klein, E., editor: Acquired immunodeficiency syndrome, Prog. Allergy **37**:1, 1986.

Matsumoto, S., et al.: Progress in primary immunodeficiency, Immunol. Today **13**:4, 1992.

Morgan, B.P., and Walport, M.J.: Complement deficiency and disease, Immunol. Today **12**:301, 1991.

Oltvai, Z.N., et al.: C1 inhibitor deficiency: molecular and immunologic basis of hereditary and acquired angioedema, Lab. Invest. **65**:381, 1991.

Rosse, W.F.: Paroxysmal nocturnal hemoglobinuria and decay accelerating factor, Annu. Rev. Med. **41**:431, 1990.

Rother, K., and Rother, U., editors: Hereditary and acquired complement deficiencies in animals and man, Prog. Allergy **39**:1, 1986.

Schultz, L.D.: Hematopoiesis and models of immunodeficiency, Semin. Immunol. **3**:397, 1991.

Case 1 A Wee Bit and Lacking

Geraldine W., a 13-day-old girl, had weighed 3560 g at birth and at that time showed no signs of illness. In the last few days she had developed a cough and was taken to a physician. Antibiotics were prescribed. Because two siblings had died of pneumonia before they were 6 months of age, the pediatrician asked the baby's mother to report every few days about her daughter's progress.

At the age of 22 days, Geraldine developed severe diarrhea with fever and had still not become free of her cough. The pediatrician was called, and he insisted on seeing the infant. During his examination of the infant, rales were noted for the first time at the base of both lungs. Geraldine now weighed 3225 g. Failure to eliminate the cough, the apparent pneumonia, the diarrhea, and the weight loss suggested a possible diagnosis of an immunodeficiency syndrome. Numerous blood studies were ordered with the following results:

	Geraldine	**Normal**
Total lymphocyte count	0.80	> 1.5
T cells (S-RBC method)	391 mm^3	2050–8000 mm^3
Expressed as percent	4%	Approximately 60%
B cells (surface IgM flow cytometry)	15%	10–20%
Response to concanavalin A	4000 cpm	25,000–120,000 cpm
Interpretation	Negative	Positive
Response to pokeweed mitogen	480 cpm	35,000–40,000 cpm
Interpretation	Positive	Positive
Nitroblue tetrazolium reductase	Normal	Normal
IgG	1.4 g/dl	1.7–8.1 g/dl
IgA	0.04 g/dl	0.2–1.0 g/dl
IgM	0.5 g/dl	0.5–0.85 g/dl

Questions

1. What is the basis of the S-RBC rosetting method for determining the T cell count?
2. What methods are used to enumerate CD4 and CD8 T cells?
3. Explain flow cytometry as used to enumerate B cells. Is this the same as FACS?
4. Describe concanavalin A and pokeweed mitogen and their applications.
5. How is the nitroblue tetrazolium reductase test performed, and what is its purpose?
6. The IgA and IgM values are much below adult levels. Explain.
7. Why is the IgG level essentially normal?
8. Are the immunoglobulin normal values presented adult normals or infant normals?
9. Defend your diagnosis of an immunoglobulin T cell or severe combined immunodeficiency.
10. What other tests would be useful to help establish your diagnosis?
11. What therapy do you recommend?

Student Questions

Case 2 A Sickly Lad

José Luis, a 6-year-old boy of Mexican inheritance, was seen by a pediatrician in the United States just 3 months after his parents had entered this country. The earlier medical history of the boy could not be established exactly, since no records were available, but his parents described José Luis as a sickly child who had numerous ear infections, pneumonia on at least two occasions, and several skin infections resembling impetigo and folliculitis. At this time, pneumonia was again diagnosed on the basis of a physical examination, which was later confirmed by x-ray. Coagulase-positive *Staphylococcus aureus* was isolated from sputum, further confirming the diagnosis.

Laboratory blood studies of the patient provided the following results:

IgG	850 mg/dl (normal)
IgM	350 mg/dl (elevated)
IgA	225 mg/dl (normal)

Normal T and B cell numbers

Normal granulocyte counts and distribution

Normal nitroblue tetrazolium reductase test after neutrophil exposure to phorbol myristate but not when exposed to latex particles

Questions

1. IgM is elevated but not the other immunoglobulins. Can you offer an explanation for this?
2. Just because T and B cell numbers are normal, does that mean lymphokine and immunoglobulin production are normal?
3. Explain the method and interpretation of the nitroblue tetrazolium reductase test.

4. What is phorbol myristate, and how does it activate neutrophils?
5. Since immunoglobulins and T and B cells are all normal, is a granulocyte deficiency the only remaining diagnosis?
6. Do any of the data suggest or eliminate a complement deficiency?
7. Doesn't the clinical history also permit the consideration of interleukin-1 (IL-1) and/or tumor necrosis factor alpha (TNF-α) secretion defects?
8. Describe the integrins and their role in immunity.
9. Do integrins and adhesins differ?
10. Describe other deficiencies of phagocytic cells that are related to diminished levels of surface components.

Student Questions

Case 3 Oh, How I Hate to Get Up in the Morning

Frank S., a 17-year-old marine recruit, awoke exhausted that morning and thought that his skin had taken on a yellow-gray pallor. He also noticed that his urine was dark yellow-brown. This was on a morning after a particularly strenuous day of mock beach attacks, so Frank wasn't particularly alarmed about these changes in view of all the stresses of boot camp. Within another day, Frank's skin and urine were returning to their normal color.

Now, 7 months later, Frank awoke one morning and delivered a dark, nearly black urine. He felt no fever, chills, or other major discomfort except some fatigue. Nevertheless, he reported to sick bay, where he appeared pale, though with a slight yellow tinge. Physical examination indicated that his spleen was tender and enlarged. Blood drawn for hematologic studies had a low hematocrit. The plasma above the cellular components was red. Further red blood cell and plasma protein studies were considered.

Questions

1. What are the major functions of the spleen?
2. What data would be agreeable with an autoimmune hemolytic disease?
3. What would a low complement C3 and normal C4 value suggest?
4. Doesn't hemolysis require both antibody and complement? Explain.
5. Discuss the concept of "standby" lysis of red cells.
6. Why have these two episodes of hemoglobinuria developed at night?
7. Discuss the modulators of complement activity.
8. Which deficiencies of the complement system lead to an increase in infections by *Neisseria*?
9. Why are deficiencies in complement molecules C1, C2, and C4 with so little influence on the incidence of bacterial infections?
10. Would you expect Frank's immunoglobulin levels to be normal?

Student Questions

Case 4 A Sickly Girl

Karen E., 3 years old, has had numerous bacterial infections. These began shortly before her first birthday and have continued until the present time. The most serious of these was a meningitis due to *Haemophilus influenzae* and two bouts of pneumonia, one due to *Staphylococcus aureus* and the other due to an unknown pathogen. Numerous visits to the pediatrician for recurrent ear infections, impetigo, and severe pharyngitis had prompted her physician to order an immunologic workup. Before this could be done, however, Karen developed a meningitis subsequently identified as due to *Serratia marcescens*. Fortunately, she recovered from this illness, and now 4 weeks later returned for the prescribed tests.

Laboratory data provided by the immunology laboratory included the following:

IgG	1100 mg/dl (elevated)
IgM	125 mg/dl (elevated)
IgA	90 mg/dl (normal)
Granulocytes	Normal numbers and distribution
Nitroblue tetrazolium reductase test	Markedly depressed
ASTO test	Elevated

Questions

1. Why are IgG and IgM considered elevated and not IgA? Are their values near adult levels?
2. What has caused the IgG and IgM values to be elevated?
3. Is the ASTO elevation related to the three identified pathogens that caused Karen's past illnesses?
4. What is the meaning of the low nitroblue tetrazolium reductase test?
5. Describe the oxidative pathway of granulocyte metabolism during phagocytosis.
6. Where does the cytochrome system fit into Karen's problem?
7. Karen's condition is often thought of as a sex-linked illness, yet she is female. Explain.
8. Describe the sex-linked immunodeficiency diseases.
9. Describe the phagocytic cell deficiency diseases.
10. Discuss the production and activity of reactive nitrogen intermediates in phagocyte-based immunity.

Student Questions

Case 5 Swelling Up but Not with Pride

Patty L., a 24-year-old graduate student in the Department of Black and Minority Studies, reported to the student health clinic with facial edema, flushing of the neck and chest, and abdominal pain. She reported that she had experienced this same phenomenon on two previous occasions in the past year. Despite efforts to identify Patty's condition as a food or inhalant allergy, an etiology could not be determined, and a diagnosis of idiopathic anaphylaxis was made.

Patty was given a prescription for an antihistamine and advised to use it at the onset of symptoms. Unfortunately, 2 months later, Patty reported to the clinic with the same symptoms despite following the recommended therapy.

Questions

1. What symptoms of anaphylaxis are consistent with those that Patty displayed?
2. What serologic tests should have been used to establish the diagnosis of idiopathic anaphylaxis more definitely?
3. Are foods commonly associated with Patty's symptomatology?
4. Describe the serocytologic basis of anaphylactic reactions.
5. Since this is apparently not a case of anaphylaxis, could it be an anaphylactoid reaction? Why or why not?
6. Complement assays of Patty's serum indicated a low hemolytic titer. What immunologic diseases does this suggest?
7. How would quantitation of C2, C3, and C4 of the complement system assist in establishing the diagnosis?
8. Because of another medical problem, danazol was given to Patty, and her edema-flushing attacks ceased. Explain.
9. In view of your answer to question 8, what other therapies are possible?

Student Questions

Review Questions

1. Chédiak-Higashi syndrome affects primarily
   A. B cells
   B. T cells
   C. NK and phagocytic cells
   D. The nitroblue tetrazolium reductase test
   E. Phagocyte mobility

2. The HIV enters T cells through the
   A. IL-2 receptor
   B. CD4 protein
   C. MHC class I protein
   D. CD3 protein
   E. Complement receptor 2

3. A deficiency in components of cytochrome b are prominent in
   A. Lazy leukocyte syndromes
   B. IgG_2 deficiency
   C. Wiskott-Aldrich syndrome
   D. Ataxia-telangiectasia
   E. Chronic granulomatous disease

4. The primary immunologic deficit in ataxia-telangiectasia is
   A. A loss of DNA repair enzymes
   B. Failure to rearrange VDJ genes of H chains
   C. Repairable with infusions of polyethylene complexed with adenosine deaminase
   D. A loss of stem cells for B lymphocytes
   E. A failure of stem B cells to mature

5. Which of the following represents a failure of B cells to mature?
   A. Chronic granulomatous disease
   B. Chronic mucocutaneous candidiasis
   C. AIDS
   D. Bruton's agammaglobulinemia
   E. Neonatal hypogammaglobulinemia

6. Which of the following is best treated with injections of extracts of lymphocytes from a healthy adult?
   A. Chronic granulomatous disease
   B. Chronic mucocutaneous candidiasis
   C. AIDS
   D. Bruton's agammaglobulinemia
   E. Neonatal hypogammaglobulinemia

7. Which of the following has no sex-linked inheritance?

A. Bruton's agammaglobulinemia
B. Wiskott-Aldrich syndrome
C. DiGeorge syndrome
D. Chronic granulomatous disease
E. None of the above

8. A lymphopenia without specification of lymphocyte type is good evidence of a deficiency of

A. NK cells
B. T cells
C. B cells
D. Lymphocytes but does not identify the cell type
E. $CD8^+$ cells

9. Tetany, which develops in a very young infant, may indicate

A. A failure of immunoglobulin switch mechanisms
B. A failure of thymic embryogenesis
C. Prenatal HIV infection
D. Bruton's agammaglobulinemia
E. None of the above

10. The ability of patients with Bruton's disease to recover normally from viral infections

A. Proves that immunoglobulins are unimportant in immunity to viral disease
B. Indicates that such patients are not totally devoid of antibody-forming capacity
C. Strongly supports a role of phagocytes in immunity to viral diseases
D. All of the above
E. None of the above

14 Transplantation Immunology

Human chromosome 6 contains the genes that encode the most important transplantation antigens (Table 14-1). These genes compose the major histocompatibility complex (MHC). The protein products of these genes are known variously as the histocompatibility, transplantation, or human leukocyte antigens (HLA). This last term is appropriate, since these antigens were first recognized as surface components of white blood cells. The dominant transplantation antigens, the class I proteins, arise from three polymorphic genes—HLA-A, HLA-B, and HLA-C. If the exact genetic assignment of an HLA antigen is uncertain, it is labeled as workshop antigen (e.g.,

Table 14-1. The human class I HLA genes and antigens

HLA-A	HLA-B	HLA-C
1	5	11 w genes
2	7	Cw1–Cw11
3	8	
9	12	
10	13	
11	14	
23	15	
24	16	
25	17	
26	18	
28	21	
29	27	
30	35	
31	37	
32	38	
Numerous w genes	39	
	40	
	44	
	45	
	49	
	Numerous w genes	

HLA-Cw8), with the expectation that a working group of experts will later determine the correct assignment. Because of the polymorphic nature of these genes, a substantial number of HLA-A, B, and C antigens are known, and it is for this reason that HLA determinations are more useful than blood grouping to identify an individual.

Since each individual has a genetic contribution from each parent, each individual has two proteins each of HLA-A, B, and C on most nucleated cells. Haplotype refers to that half of a person's genotype derived from one parent. Haplotype is determined by identifying the HLA proteins on a person's lymphocytes and the lymphocytes of one or both parents by using antibodies specific for these proteins.

The class II genes of the MHC also determine, in part, the outcome of tissue transplantation. These D region genes—DP, DQ, and DR—also encode cell surface proteins.

Class III genes of the MHC encode proteins C2, C4, and factor B of the complement system and do not govern the success or failure of tissue transplantation.

The class I proteins are 45,000 molecular weight members of the immunoglobulin gene superfamily. The class I protein is always associated with the beta$_2$-microglobulin (12,500 MW), which, because of its structural identity between persons, does not regulate transplantation success.

Because of the large number of alleles at the MHC gene loci, an exact or full antigen match of the class I antigens between a transplant donor and recipient is nearly impossible. Exceptions to this include identical twins and occasionally family members such as two siblings. Since most tissue transplants are made across an immunologic barrier, it is important to select a donor who has as near an antigen match with the recipient as possible. The microcytotoxicity test can be used for this purpose. Antisera specific for the transplant antigens are incubated with lymphocytes of the donor and recipient in the presence of complement in the microcytotoxicity test. Cell damage is determined for each antibody-cell mixture, and the HLA formula for each of the transplantation partners is thus established. An alternate method to determine histocompatibility is to measure the recipient's lymphocyte response to killed donor lymphocytes in cultures (one-way mixed leukocyte or mixed lymphocyte culture or reaction [MLC or MLR]). This is generally believed to measure the recipient T cell response to D region proteins on donor B cells.

Because a full HLA match between donor and recipient is statistically difficult to achieve, it is usually necessary to treat the transplant recipient with an immunosuppressant such as a corticosteroid, a purine, pyrimidine or folic acid analog, antilymphocyte serum, cyclosporine, or other agents that depress the T cell response. Normally several of these are incorporated into the suppressant regimen. Cytotoxic T cells are considered to be the main aggressors in graft rejection, and all of the reagents listed have an anti–T cell activity. Rejection of grafts by the recipient's preformed antibodies to the ABO blood group antigens occurs very rapidly (hyperacute rejection), but blood group antigens are not considered as transplant antigens. Graft rejection in blood group–matched individuals who are not fully HLA matched is highly dependent on T cells and is a much slower process than hyperacute rejection. Caution should be exercised when lymphoid tissue is transplanted into an immunodepressed recipient for fear of causing graft-versus-host disease (GVHD).

Certain tissues such as cornea can be successfully transplanted across the HLA barrier. The developing fetus may also be considered as a privileged tissue (or as present in a privileged site), since it is only a half match with its mother.

The relationship of MHC genes to autoimmunity is described in Chapter 7.

Key Words and Phrases

Acute rejection
Alkylating agent
Allograft
Antilymphocyte globulin (serum)
Autograft
Beta$_2$-microglobulin
Bone marrow purging
Cadaver graft
Chronic rejection
Colony-stimulating factors
Corticosteroid
Cyclophilin
Cyclophosphamide
Cyclosporine
Folic acid analog
Genotype
Graft-versus-host disease
Haplotype
Histocompatibility antigen
Hyperacute rejection
Immune enhancement
Immunotoxin
Interferon
MHC class I protein
MHC class II protein
Microcytotoxicity test
Mixed lymphocyte reaction
Privileged site
Privileged tissue
Purine analog
Pyrimidine analog
Stem cell grafting
Transplantation antigen

Abbreviations

ADCC
ALS
CTL
DP, DQ, and DR
G-CSF
GM-CSF
GVHD
HLA-A, B, and C
IFN-α
M-CSF
MLC
MLR
NK cells
TNF-β

Information Sources

Books

Baumgartner, W.A., Reitz, B.A., and Achuff, S.C., editors: Heart and heart-lung transplantation, W.B. Saunders Co., 1990, Philadelphia.

Brent, L., and Sells, R.A., editors: Organ transplantation, Bailliere Tindall, 1989, London.

Burakoff, S.J., et al., editors: Graft-vs.-host disease: immunology, pathology, and treatment, Marcel Dekker, Inc., 1990, New York.

Milford, E.L., editor: Renal transplantation, Churchill Livingstone, 1989, New York.

Pusey, C.D., editor: Immunobiology of renal disease, Kluwer Academic Publishers, 1991, Dordrecht.

Sale, G.E., editor: The pathology of organ transplantation, Butterworth, 1990, Boston.

Srivastava, R., Ram, B.P., and Tyle, P., editors: Immunogenetics of the major histocompatibility complex, VCH Publishers, 1990, New York.

Wallace, K.H., and Thompson, R.A.: Immunointervention in man, Oxford University Press, 1992, New York.

Wallwork, J., editor: Heart and heart-lung transplantation, W.B. Saunders Co., 1989, Philadelphia.

Williams, J.W., editor: Hepatic transplantation, W.B. Saunders Co., 1990, Philadelphia.

Reviews

Jadus, M.R., and Wepsec, H.T.: The role of cytokines in graft-versus-host reactions and disease, Bone Marrow Transplant. **10**:1, 1992

Roberts, J.P.: Liver transplantation today, Annu. Rev. Med. **40**:287, 1989.

Schreiber, S.L., and Crabtree, G.R.: The mechanism of action of cyclosporine A and FK 506, Immunol. Today **13**:136, 1992.

Trulock, E.P.: Lung transplantation, Annu. Rev. Med. **43**:1, 1992.

Yu, Y.Y., Kumar, V., and Bennett, M.: Murine natural killer cells and marrow graft rejection, Annu. Rev. Immunol. **10**:189, 1992.

Case 1 No Match this Time

Roger W., a 51-year-old retired tennis star, was referred to the oncology unit at University Hospital with the provisional diagnosis of chronic myelogenous leukemia. His personal physician had arranged the referral following Roger's complaint of unusual bruising and had determined that Roger had a massive splenomegaly and a white blood cell count of 250,000/mm^3. In the hospital, Roger failed to respond to interferon therapy and was eventually scheduled for an allogenic bone marrow transplantation. Roger's HLA profile was HLA-A1, A10, B7, B18, Cw1-D; region proteins were not determined.

Subsequently Roger received total body irradiation and high-dose therapy with cytosine arabinoside and cyclophosphamide. Two days thereafter, he received bone marrow from a mismatched donor whose HLA composition was A3, A9, B7, B8, Cw2, Cw3. Within 10 days, a severe graft-versus-host reaction was observed, and Roger was treated with a monoclonal anti-CD8-ricin conjugate. His response was remarkable, and 15 days later on April 6, he was discharged.

Roger was hopeful that he would be able to attend the U.S. Open Tennis Tournament as a spectator, but in August, exactly 90 days after his discharge, Roger was readmitted with GVHD. His condition deteriorated steadily despite intermittent high-dose therapy with a glucocorticoid. Ten months and 2 days after his first admission to the hospital, Roger expired.

Questions

1. Describe the interferons—their source, mode of action, and use in therapy of chronic myelogenous leukemia.
2. What is the meaning of the terms *half mismatch, quarter mismatch,* and so on in relation to HLA and transplantation?
3. How are monoclonal immunotoxins prepared, and how do they function?
4. What are the immunologic findings of GVHD?
5. What is the role of steroid therapy in GVHD?
6. How would a stem cell graft avoid some of the problems Roger encountered?
7. Why was CD8 chosen as the antigen target of the passive immunization?
8. For what immunoproliferative conditions is bone marrow transplantation recommended?
9. In a similar case, an anti-CD15-ricin conjugate was used. Why was this chosen rather than anti-CD8?
10. Explain the use and potential benefit of colony-stimulating factor therapy in bone marrow transplantation.

Student Questions

Case 2 A Lucky Stiff

David L., a 36-year-old employee of the Internal Revenue Service, had suffered from bad health the past 8 years. In the beginning, this consisted of spontaneous, temporary feverish episodes during which no infectious disease could be identified. Edema of both ankles usually accompanied the fever, but the accompanying extreme fatigue persisted after the fever and edema had disappeared. On several occasions, David sought medical advice, but a diagnosis was never established.

At age 32, David had suffered a bout of extreme abdominal pain in the lower left quadrant that prompted his hospitalization. Because data from urinalysis were abnormal, a kidney biopsy was taken. A diagnosis of glomerulonephritis with fibrosis and tubular degeneration was made at that time.

Now, 4 years later, total kidney failure was diagnosed, and hemodialysis was initiated. David had no brothers or sisters, and his mother had died 12 years earlier of "uremic poisoning." The inability to locate David's father led to the conclusion that a close HLA match would be difficult to find, and because of David's condition, a kidney cadaver transplant was performed.

Post-transplant graft maintenance was attempted with azathioprine (100 mg/day) and prednisolone (25 mg/day). Kidney function remained normal for 3 months, at which time a slight loss in function became apparent. Accordingly, prednisolone was increased to 50 mg/day. Roger's kidney function quickly returned to normal.

Reexamination of the kidney biopsy originally diagnosed as glomerulonephritic was consistent with a diagnosis of Fabry's disease.

Questions

1. What is a half HLA match between donor and recipient?
2. Why wasn't HLA typing done in this case?
3. Can one expect, by chance, a half match for cadaver grafts?
4. Is HLA matching less important in predicting kidney survival than it is for other tissues?
5. What would the findings be for a glomerulonephritis of immune origin?
6. What is the basis of the immunosuppressive activity of azathioprine?
7. What is the basis of the immunosuppressive activity of prednisolone?
8. What other immunosuppressants would you consider in addition to cyclosporine?
9. What is cyclosporine?
10. What is cyclophilin?

Student Questions

Case 3 Hepatitis Aftermath

John W., the 12-year-old son of a navy officer, was admitted to the Public Health Hospital with a diagnosis of viral hepatitis on August 7, 1970. In addition, and as the result of additional findings—hemoglobin of 12 mg/dl, platelet count of 6000/mm^3, and white cell count of 900/mm^3—he was diagnosed to have a pancytopenia, probably aplastic anemia associated with the hepatitis. At this time, tests for Australia antigen were negative. Red cell and platelet transfusions were given immediately. Although John's liver function tests improved daily, his blood cell profile remained critical, usually having less than 5% granulocytes.

During the next 2 weeks, bouts of streptococcal meningitis and gram-negative bacterial septicemia were combatted successfully with antibiotics. On day 17, after admission, a bone marrow graft from an HLA class I–identical, blood group–identical sister was performed. The MLC assay could not be done for lack of recipient marrow. Methotrexate, 6 mg/m^2 of body surface, and antilymphocyte serum (equine) were begun. The latter was given on two occasions, 6 days apart, and withdrawn from the regimen after the second injection.

On day 42 after the bone marrow transplant, John developed an erythematous rash over his chest and extremities compatible with GVHD. The methotrexate dose was increased to 10 mg/m^2, and over the following days the rash disappeared. Shortly thereafter, a vesicular eruption appeared on the left side of the abdomen consistent with that of a herpes zoster infection. This was still creating considerable discomfort when John was discharged 61 days after the bone marrow transplant.

Questions

1. Why aren't granulocyte transfusions or white blood cell transfusions applied in this case?
2. Isn't there a role for colony-stimulating factors in cases like John's?
3. Diagram a hypothetical class I MHC haplotype for John's two parents, himself, and his sister.
4. Describe variations of MLC assays.
5. How are antilymphocyte serum and globulin prepared?
6. How is the potency of antilymphocyte serum determined?
7. Why is antilymphocyte serum withdrawn from post-transplant surgery in most instances?
8. Discuss the mode of action of methotrexate.
9. How can GVHD develop in class I MHC–matched donor and recipient?
10. What viral and other infectious risks accompany immunosuppressive therapy of transplant patients?

Student Questions

Case 4 A Good Outcome

Bryan M., a 57-year-old victim of kidney failure, was now being prepared for his kidney graft. Over the past several years, he had received numerous blood transfusions before and during the time he was on hemodialysis. His HLA-A, B, and C antigen makeup had been identified months ago. The transplant team confirmed the earlier results of this typing and extended this to the DR antigens by the microcytotoxicity test. Bryan was HLA-A1, A9, B8, B27, Cw3, Cw4, DR1, DR9 and blood group A. The donor was also blood group A and represented an HLA half match for A, B, C, and DR. Since DP and DQ antigens had not been assayed, an MLC was arranged, even though the results would not be available until after the transplant had been accomplished.

After the transplant, Bryan passed 3.6 liters of urine the first day, and the urea and creatinine levels indicated near normal kidney function. The standard immunosuppressant regimen used by the transplant team was continued for 7 days, after which only a corticosteroid was administered.

Four months later, Bryan continued in good health with no rejection episodes.

Questions

1. Describe the chemistry of the HLA-A, B, and C antigens.
2. Describe the chemistry of the D region proteins.
3. What is the influence of multiple blood transfusions on graft acceptance?
4. How is the microcytotoxicity test conducted and interpreted?
5. How could you determine Bryan's haplotypes?
6. How is the MLC assay conducted and interpreted?
7. How can one shorten the time needed to achieve results in MLC assays?
8. Describe cyclophilin and cyclosporin.
9. What is a one-way MLC assay?

Student Questions

Review Questions

1. Which of the following antigens controlled by genes of the MHC does not function as a transplantation barrier?
   A. HLA-A
   B. HLA-B
   C. DP
   D. Complement C4
   E. HLA-C

2. Hyperacute graft rejection is associated with
   A. Antibodies to ABO antigens in the donor tissue
   B. A second graft from an individual who donated the first graft
   C. Preformed antibodies to antigens in the donated tissue
   D. All of the above
   E. Only answers A and C

3. Which of the following children is/are HLA incompatible with the two adults?

Adult male	A1, A2, B8, B12, Cw-, Cw6
Adult female	A3, A9, B5, B7, Cw3, Cw6
Child 1	A1, A9, B7, B8, Cw3, Cw6
Child 2	A1, A3, B5, B12, Cw-, Cw6
Child 3	A1, A2, B5, B12; Cw3, Cw6

   A. Child 1
   B. Child 2
   C. Child 3
   D. Children 1 and 2
   E. Children 1 and 3

4. In which of the following is graft-versus-host disease (GVHD) most apt to occur?

A. Lymphoid tissue transplant to an immunodeficient recipient
B. Transplantation of skin between allogenically different individuals
C. Transplantation of irradiated lymphoid tissue across the histocompatibility barrier
D. Transplantation of fetal tissue to an adult
E. Allogenic transplantation of any kind

5. Which of the following agents has the $CD4^+$ T cell as a major target?

A. Prednisolone
B. Cyclosporine
C. Antilymphocyte serum
D. Methotrexate
E. Azathioprine

6. Purging of bone marrow prior to transplantation may be of value if it

A. Kills NK cells in the marrow
B. Removes $CD8^+$ cells from the marrow
C. Deletes leukemic cells from the marrow
D. Uses monoclonal antibodies against T lymphocytes in the marrow
E. All of the above

7. Genes of the MHC encode all of the following except

A. Genes of the person's haplotype
B. Class I proteins
C. $Beta_2$ microglobulin
D. D region genes
E. Complement

8. A concern of immunosuppressive treatment of a transplant recipient is

A. The inability to resist an infectious disease
B. Possible GVHD when lymphoid tissue is transplanted
C. The emergency of a neoplasm
D. The appearance of a latent viral infection
E. All of the above

9. Which of the following has traditionally been considered a privileged tissue in transplantation immunology?

A. The developing fetus
B. Erythrocytes
C. $CD4^-8^-$ lymphocytes
D. Kidney
E. Bone marrow

10. Which of the following has the longest expected survival?

A. Heart transplant from a baboon to a human
B. Human-to-human heart transplant
C. Human-to-human kidney transplant
D. Human-to-baboon liver transplant
E. Human-to-human liver transplant

15 Tumor Immunology

Antigenic changes normally accompany the biochemical, morphologic, and genetic alterations associated with the appearance of the neoplastic cells. The extent of these antigenic adjustments varies considerably from one situation to another and, in fact, is unpredictable for chemically induced tumors. Virus-induced tumors produce two types of antigens—those of the virus itself and the new cancer cell antigens. The latter are antigenically constant for any virus-host relationship. New antigens on cancer cells are designated as tumor-associated antigens (TAA), tumor-specific antigens (TSA), or tumor-specific transplantation antigens (TSTA). Tumor-associated antigen refers to any antigen associated with the carcinogenic state. This could even be a viral antigen in virus-induced tumors. Tumor-specific antigen refers to an antigen associated with a specific cancer but not encountered in other types of cancer or on normal cells, although this latter criterion has been difficult to prove. Tumor-specific transplantation antigens are surface antigens novel to tumor cells that under the proper circumstances would stimulate tumor autograft rejection even in an otherwise syngeneic animal. Oncofetal (carcinofetal) antigens are those produced by an embryonic tissue and by that same tissue when it becomes cancerous in an adult. Traces of these oncofetal antigens are often present in healthy cancer-free adults, and certain non-neoplastic, inflammatory states may also stimulate oncofetal antigen production. Titration of the blood level of these antigens, such as carcinoembryonic antigen (CEA), assists in the diagnosis of cancer and is useful in evaluating cancer therapy.

Neoplastic growth of lymphocytes and other cells that participate in the immune response are of special interest to immunologists (Table 15-1). Multiple myeloma, a proliferation of mature B cells, can be either monoclonal, in which case a single B cell line has become transformed, or polyclonal, in which several lines of B cells have become neoplastic. The clonality of multiple myeloma can be determined on occasion by the appearance of a single or of multiple immunoglobulin peaks, known as the M (myeloma) components, in the immunoelectrophoretic profile of the serum. Waldenström's macroglobulinemia refers to neoplasia of IgM-producing cells; in multiple myeloma, other gamma globulins are affected. In some cases, excess, free κ or λ light chains (Bence Jones proteins) in blood and urine are indicative of the B lymphocyte abnormality.

Non-T acute lymphocytic leukemia (non-T-ALL) is essentially equivalent to B-cell leukemia and is only one of several varieties of leukemia. In Burkitt's lymphoma, another B cell disease, interesting chromosomal translocations move the cellular *myc* gene to either chromosome 14, 2, or 22, the chromosomes where H, κ, and λ chain genes reside. In nasopharyngeal carcinoma, these same translocations occur. It is

Table 15-1. Selected cancers of lymphocytic cells

B cell conditions
Acute lymphocytic leukemia (B-ALL)
Chronic lymphocytic leukemia
Hairy cell leukemia
Waldenström's macroglobulinemia
Multiple myeloma
Burkitt's lymphoma
T cell conditions
Acute lymphocytic leukemia (T-ALL)
Chronic lymphocytic anemia
Cutaneous T-cell leukemia (Sézary syndrome)
NK cell conditions
NK cell leukemia

believed that this places the *myc* oncogene under control of immunoglobulin promoters as an essential step in the development of these two cancers. It is interesting that an Epstein-Barr virus infection is associated with both of these neoplasms. Burkitt's lymphoma cells are B cells at an early stage of development. Hairy cell leukemia affects more adult B cells near the level of those recognized in Waldenström's macroglobulinemia.

T-cell acute leukemias (T-ALL) can be identified by rearrangements in the TCR genes if other surface markers, the CD proteins, cannot be used. Chronic lymphocytic leukemia is characterized by excessive $CD8^+$ suppressor T cell production and cutaneous T-cell leukemia by $CD4^+$ helper T cell proliferation. Lymphocytes seen in Hodgkin's disease are known for their variability from one patient to another, preventing a clear-cut classification. NK-cell leukemia is also known.

Cells in the myeloid series may also become neoplastic, as in chronic myelogenous leukemia.

How tumor cells with their antigenic differences from normal cells escape the immune surveillance system is unclear. Antigen modulation and immune suppression are two of the most plausible theories.

Several avenues of potential immunotherapy of cancer have been tested, but unfortunately the success has only been marginal in most instances. A few successes can be cited, however. Stimulation of macrophages by BCG vaccination is occasionally successful and is recommended for bladder cancer. Activated macrophages secrete tumor necrosis factor alpha (TNF-α). BCG also activates NK, T, and B cells. Recently interferon alpha (IFN-α) has been licensed for treatment of hairy cell leukemia and chronic myelogenous leukemia. Immunotoxins—tumor-specific antibodies conjugated to cell toxins (diphtheria toxin, for example)—are still in the experimental stage as therapeutic agents but have had application in bone marrow purging. The expansion of peripheral blood lymphocytes from cancer patients or of lymphocytes harvested from tumors by exposure to interleukin-1 (IL-1), IL-2, and IFN-α in culture has provided unique cell populations for adoptive immunization of these patients. These cells are known as LAK (lymphokine-activated killer) cells and TILs (tumor-infiltrating lymphocytes), respectively. In the future, bifunctional antibodies may have a role in cancer therapy.

Key Words and Phrases

Terms from genetics, virology, and cellular and molecular biology appear frequently in the vocabulary of tumor immunology.

Adjuvant therapy
Alpha-fetoprotein
Antigenic modulation
Bacille Calmette-Guérin
Bence Jones protein
Bifunctional antibody
Burkitt's lymphoma
Carcinoembryonic antigen
Carcinofetal antigen
Chromosomal translocation
Common acute lymphocytic leukemia antigen
Condyloma acuminatum
Epstein-Barr virus
Hairy cell leukemia
Hepatitis B virus
Herpes virus
Hodgkin's disease
Immune surveillance
Immune enhancement
Immunoimaging
Immunoscintigraphy
Immunotoxin
Lymphocytic leukemia
M component
Multiple myeloma
Nasopharyngeal carcinoma
Natural killer cell
Oncofetal antigen
Oncogene
Papilloma virus
Plasmacytoma
Proto-oncogene
Tumor-associated antigen
Tumor-specific antigen
Tumor-specific transplantation antigen
Waldenström's macroglobulinemia

Abbreviations

AFP
ALL
B-ALL
BCG
CALLA
CEA
CML
EBV
HIV
HTLV-I
HTLV-II
IFN-α and γ
IL-2
LAK
NK cell
TAA
T-ALL
TIL
TNF-α
TSA
TSTA

Information Sources

Books

Balkwill, F.R.: Cytokines in cancer therapy, Oxford University Press, 1989, New York.

Beutler, B., editor: Tumor necrosis factors, Raven Press, Inc., 1992, New York.

deKermon, J.B., editor: Immunotherapy of urological tumors, Churchill Livingstone, 1990, Edinburgh.

Lotzova, E., and Herberman, R.B., editors: Immunobiology of natural killer cells, CRC Press, Inc., 1986, Boca Raton.

Magerstadt, M.: Antibody conjugates and malignant disease, CRC Press, Inc., 1991, Boca Raton.

Osawa, T., and Bonavida, B., editors: Tumor necrosis factor: structure-function relationship and clinical application, S. Karger AG, 1992, Basel.

Perkins, A.C., and Pimm, M.V.: Immunoscintigraphy: Practical aspects and clinical applications, Wiley-Liss, Inc., 1991, New York.

Wallace, K.H., and Thompson, R.A.: Immunointervention in man, Oxford University Press, 1992, New York.

Wallace, K.H., and Thompson, R.A.: The natural killer cell, IRL Press, 1992, Oxford.

Reviews

Jacobs, E.L., and Haskell, C.M.: Clinical use of tumor markers in oncology, Curr. Prob. Cancer **15**:299, 1992.

Kluin-Nelemans, H.: Hairy cell leukemia and its T cell interactions, Leukemia Lymphoma **4**:159, 1991.

LoBuglio, A.F., and Saleh, M.N.: Monoclonal antibody therapy in cancer, Crit. Rev. Oncol. Hematol. **13**:271, 1992.

Matutes, E., and Catovsky, D.: Mature T cell leukemias and leukemia/lymphoma syndromes, Leukemia Lymphoma **4**:81, 1991.

Melief, C.J.: Tumor eradication by adoptive transfer of cytotoxic T lymphocytes, Adv. Cancer Res. **58**:143, 1992.

Neville, A.M.: Detection of tumor antigens with monoclonal antibodies: immunopathology and immunodiagnosis, Curr. Opin. Immunol. **3**:674, 1991.

Oettgen, H.F.: Cytokines in clinical cancer therapy, Curr. Opin. Immunol. **3**:699, 1991.

Pardoll, D.: New strategies for active immunotherapy with genetically engineered tumor cells, Curr. Opin. Immunol. **4**:619, 1992.

Ramakrishnan, S.: Current status of antibody-toxin conjugates for tumor therapy, Targeted Diagn. Ther. **3**:189, 1990.

Vaickus, L.: Immune markers in hematologic malignancies, Crit. Rev. Oncol. Hematol. **11**:267, 1991.

Whiteside, T.L., Jost, L.M., and Herberman, R.B.: Tumor infiltrating lymphocytes: potential and limitations to their use for cancer therapy, Crit. Rev. Oncol. Hematol. **12**:25, 1992.

Case 1 Time Did Tell

Seven-year-old Cayle B., a victim of a T-cell lymphoma, was being prepared for an autologous bone marrow graft. Previously collected bone marrow was treated with a mixture of monoclonal antibodies specific for CD1, CD2, CD5, and CD7 plus complement. As conditioning for reengraftment, Cayle received total body irradiation and cyclophosphamide, 120 mg/m^2 of body surface. Two days later, Cayle received the purged bone marrow (1.4×10^4 granulocyte-monocyte colony-forming units/kg of body weight).

On day 15 after receiving the bone marrow, Cayle's peripheral blood lymphocytes consisted of 50% CD8 and 35% CD57 positive cells. Nearly 22% of the lymphocytes were dually positive for these markers. Subsequently, Cayle received an infusion of monoclonal murine anti-CD8, 0.2 mg/kg/day in two divided doses, daily for 6 days. Cayle showed no untoward reaction to this antiserum.

Fifteen days later, Cayle's lymphocyte profile consisted of 20% CD8 and 14% CD57 cells with 4% being dually positive. After an additional 2 weeks, the granulocyte and platelet counts, which were both depressed 15 days post-transplant, became normal.

Now, approximately 1 year after engraftment, peripheral blood granulocyte and platelet counts remain normal. CD8 and CD4 cells represent 20% and 40%, respectively, of the lymphocytes.

Questions

1. What is the specificity of the monoclonal antibodies specific for CD1, CD2, CD5, and CD7?
2. Discuss the chemistry and mode of action of cyclophosphamide.
3. Why was there a 2-day delay after cyclophosphamide therapy before the bone marrow was reinfused?
4. Describe alternative methods of purging autologous bone marrow.
5. Which cells are CD8 positive, and which are CD57 positive? What do these markers represent?
6. Explain the nature of the cells that are both CD8 and CD57 positive.
7. Why was anti-CD8 administered, and why for only 6 days?
8. Is 20% CD8 and 14% CD57 an abnormal or normal reading? Explain.
9. Is 20% CD8 and 40% CD4 a normal or abnormal reading?
10. Why weren't granulocyte or platelet transfusions attempted early after the transplantation?

Student Questions

Case 2 She Had a Nose for It

Jian H., a 28-year-old physician from South China, was in San Francisco to begin 3 years of postgraduate study. About 3 months after her arrival in the United States, she began to notice fullness and discomfort in her right ear. As a physician, she made her own differential diagnosis and consulted with a colleague in the EENT Division of the Department of Surgery for confirmation. Her friend's physical examination revealed that Jian had a mass in the posterior right nasal space involving the eustachian cushion. A biopsy of this mass was identified histologically as a nasopharyngeal carcinoma. Jian was treated with cyclophosphamide, 750 mg/m^2, and doxorubicin, 50 mgm/m^2, on a 3-week cycle for nine cycles.

At the present time, Jian is disease free and in the second year of postgraduate study.

Questions

1. Nasopharyngeal carcinoma is highly limited to the Southeast Asian Chinese. What is the explanation for this?
2. C structure and/or "donuts" in cells of nasopharyngeal cancer have been identified as viral structures. Discuss.
3. What viruses are associated with human malignancies?
4. How is nasopharyngeal carcinoma related to Burkitt's lymphoma?
5. Describe the chromosomal translocations observed in Burkitt's lymphoma.
6. Compare cellular oncogenes (proto-oncogenes) with viral oncogenes.
7. Discuss oncogene products as they relate to cell transformation.
8. What type of lymphocytes are involved in Burkitt's lymphoma?
9. Are Burkitt's cells or those of nasopharyngeal carcinoma generally sensitive to therapy with cyclophosphamide and/or doxorubicin?

Student Questions

Case 3 A Partially Cultured Person

Laurel C., a 37-year-old self-employed manager of a small housecleaning firm, had been diagnosed to have hepatocellular carcinoma. Alpha-fetoprotein assays had been used to establish the diagnosis in addition to immunoscintigraphy. Laurel volunteered to enter an experimental therapeutic trial, which was carefully explained to her.

Peripheral blood lymphocytes were harvested from Laurel by leukophoresis and gradient purification. The cells at 3×10^6/ml were placed in a growth medium that contained 4 units/ml of recombinant interleukin-2 (rIL-2) and maintained in culture for 5 days. The cultures were harvested and washed, and 2×10^9 cells were infused into an intrahepatic artery. This was repeated 1 week later, although the cell population this time was slightly greater, 4.2×10^9 cells.

Immediately after the first injection of the cultured cells, 1200 U/day of rIL-2 was given by intramuscular injection and repeated later that day. This regimen was continued daily for 3 weeks until side effects could no longer be controlled by indomethacin, at which time rIL-2 therapy was terminated.

Although Laurel's alpha-fetoprotein level diminished significantly during therapy, it again became elevated. Laurel is now scheduled for a second course of therapy, which will include the addition of a bifunctional antibody.

Questions

1. Describe alpha-fetoprotein—its origin, chemistry, and use in cancer diagnosis.
2. What other markers are useful in the diagnosis of hepatocellular carcinoma?
3. Compare the history of carcinoembryonic agent (CEA) and alpha-fetoprotein in cancer diagnosis and prognosis.
4. What noncancerous conditions elevate the blood level of alpha-fetoprotein?
5. Describe rIL-2 and its receptor.
6. How is the biologic activity of IL-2 determined?
7. What are the side effects of IL-2 therapy?
8. How do LAK cells and TIL cells differ?
9. Describe immunoscintigraphy.
10. Discuss bifunctional antibodies and their potential role in cancer therapy.

Student Questions

Case 4 A Two-Time Loser

Arthur M., a 67-year-old retiree, presented himself for one of his regularly scheduled urologic examinations. These had been necessary the past 4 years because of two urologic problems. Four years ago, at Arthur's routine annual physical examination, an enlarged prostate was discovered. Subsequent laboratory tests revealed a high prostate-specific antigen (PSA) level. Histologic examination of a prostate biopsy was inconclusive regarding the possibility of prostatic cancer. On that basis, prostate resection and castration were both rejected, and PSA titrations were included with the physical examinations every 6 months.

Two years after this experience, an episode of hematuria led Arthur to believe that another form of prostate trouble had befallen him. Urologic and histologic examination, however, identified a transitional cell carcinoma on the bladder wall, which was then surgically removed. Frequent examinations over these past 2 years revealed several recurrences of bladder cancer. In each case, the growth was surgically removed. At this time, Arthur's urologist advised intravesicular BCG immunization.

Questions

1. What is prostate-specific antigen?
2. With what confidence can PSA titers be used to diagnose the presence or predict the prognosis of prostatic cancer?
3. What immunotherapeutic possibilities exist for prostatic cancer?
4. What is the past history of BCG vaccination in cancer therapy?
5. How would the results of PPD skin test affect the choice of BCG vaccination?
6. What immunoreactive cells are influenced by BCG immunization, and what are the cancer-controlling products formed by these cells?
7. The side effects of BCG immunization have been partially controlled by isoniazid. What is the influence of this on BCG immunization?
8. BCG vaccination has been used to treat melanoma in the past. What is the present status of this?
9. What is the prospect of immunization against chemically induced or viral-related cancers?

Student Questions

Review Questions

1. Burkitt's lymphoma is associated with
   A. A chromosome 8/14 translocation
   B. Movement of a c-*myc* gene near to a promoter gene
   C. Epstein-Barr virus infection
   D. Similar events as seen in nasopharyngeal carcinoma
   E. All of the above

2. Viruses associated with tumor formation in humans include
   A. Hepatitis B virus
   B. Epstein-Barr virus
   C. Papilloma viruses
   D. Retroviruses
   E. All of the above

3. Immunoscintigraphy is defined as
   A. A form of immunotherapy
   B. The use of an immunotoxin in tumor therapy
   C. A diagnostic procedure for radioimaging cancers
   D. A serologic test similar to RIA methods
   E. Answers A, B, and C

4. Oncofetal antigen
   A. Synthesis stops at birth in healthy individuals
   B. Titration is often valuable in evaluating cancer therapy
   C. Formation follows infection with oncogenic viruses
   D. Synthesis is limited to cancers of the intestinal tract and associated tissues
   E. Cannot be detected in blood by immunodiffusion assays

5. A tumor-specific transplantation antigen (TSTA) is
   A. An antigen present on the surface of a tumor cell not found on normal cells
   B. The same as a tumor-associated antigen (TAA)
   C. An antigen produced by a tumor cell as the result of viral infection
   D. Any antigen present on a tumor cell surface
   E. Simply the increased concentration of a normal antigen produced by tumor cells

6. The mode of action of BCG vaccine in tumor therapy is related to its
   A. Induction of $CD8^+$ T cells that attack the tumor directly
   B. Activation of granulocytes
   C. Ability to stimulate T_H cells and thereby antibody synthesis
   D. Activation of macrophages
   E. Ability to halt blocking antibody formation

7. Which of the following is **not** considered as a neoplasm of B lymphocytes?

A. Hairy cell leukemia
B. Waldenström's macroglobulinemia
C. Sézary syndrome (cutaneous leukemia)
D. Multiple myeloma
E. Burkitt's lymphoma

8. Interferon alpha (INF-α) is approved for the treatment

A. Of all carcinoembryonic-producing tumors
B. Chronic myelogenous leukemia
C. Breast cancer
D. Lung cancer
E. Melanoma

9. A polyclonal gammopathy

A. Is the result of neoplasia in several lines of B cells
B. Is detectable by excessive production of more than one immunoglobulin
C. May also be associated with the presence of Bence Jones protein in urine
D. May be reflected by the appearance of Russell bodies in plasma cells
E. All of the above

10. Hodgkin's disease is

A. A malignancy of T cells
B. Often cured by therapy
C. A malignancy of myeloid cells
D. Usually treated with TILs
E. Usually treated with LAK cells

16 Autoimmunity

When effector components of the immune system become directed at self-targets, an autoimmune disease may develop, although limited self-directed expressions of this type are considered normal. Self-directed T cells and immunoglobulins may not be the initiators of autoimmune diseases whose etiology is often unknown, but their activities often perpetuate the disease. The identification of these misbehaving cells or antibodies is often useful in the diagnosis of these diseases.

A variety of immunologic events are associated with autoimmune diseases. These diseases may appear because of errors in immune recognition or immune regulation. The failure of immune regulation in systemic lupus erythematosus (SLE) is evidenced by a decrease in the suppressor T cell population, which subsequently allows an undesired autoantibody to be formed. In insulin-dependent diabetes mellitus, an untoward number of major histocompatibility complex (MHC) class II antigen presenting cells may be initiators of the disease.

Unusual antigen relationships are also related to some autoimmune conditions. Common cross-reactive antigens present in certain group A streptococci and the human heart permit the immune response to these bacteria to cause post-streptococcal rheumatic fever. Antigen mimicry of this type has also been recognized in post-streptococcal glomerulonephritis. The recently identified stress or heat shock proteins, which have an antigenic commonality between microbial and mammalian cells, may also be participants in the development of autoimmune disease. New epitopes created by chemical (haptenic) additions to host proteins are the immunologic origin of idiopathic thrombocytopenic purpura and a few other diseases. Failure of an individual to recognize self-molecules as self (self-tolerance), instead treating them as foreign antigens, is characteristic of some autoimmune diseases, especially those where these molecules are not synthesized until after the immune system has matured.

The genetic influence on the immune response is founded in the genes and proteins of the MHC class II complex. In several instances, an exact DP, DQ, or DR gene can be associated with an autoimmune disease in a mathematical relationship known as relative risk (Table 16-1). Even when a class II gene association is difficult, a class I MHC relationship may be detectable, particularly with HLA-B genes which are the class I genes positioned nearest to class II genes. The relative risk (RR) calculation for ankylosing spondylitis and the class I B27 antigen is 90. Other RR values are usually lower but still provide insights into the genetic basis of these autoimmune diseases.

Another aspect of autoimmunity, the identification of the key antigens involved in each disease, has captured the attention of the molecular immunologists (Table 16-2). Surprisingly the early identification of a receptor as the major antigen in Graves'

Table 16-1. Relative risk calculations for a selection of autoimmune diseases

Disease	Relative risk	HLA antigen
Ankylosing spondylitis	90	B27
Reiter's syndrome	36	B27
Insulin-dependent diabetes mellitus	33	DR3/4
Celiac disease	11.2	B8
Myasthenia gravis	4.5	B8
Systemic lupus erythematosus	3	DR2

Table 16-2. Autoimmune diseases classified by immune target

Disease	Antigen involved	Antibody/T cell involvement
RECEPTOR TARGET		
Graves' disease	Receptor for thyotropin-stimulating hormone	LATS (long-acting thyroid stimulator), an antibody that activates the receptor
Myasthenia gravis	Acetylcholine receptor	Antibodies block reaction of receptor with acetylcholine
CROSS-REACTING ANTIGEN		
Post-streptococcal glomerulonephritis	Several M proteins (e.g., 5, 12, 18, 49, 53) of group A streptococci	Antibody to streptococcal lipoprotein cross reacts with kidney
Post-streptococcal rheumatic fever	Numerous M protein types of group A streptococci	Antibody to a common sequence on M proteins cross reacts with cardiac myosin
Ankylosing spondylitis	HLA-B27	Antibody to enzyme of *Klebsiella* bacteria cross reacts with HLA-27
ENZYME ANTIGEN		
Systemic lupus erythematosus	dsDNA, snRNP, U family of ribozymes	Antibody, loss of T_s cells noted
Polymyositis	tRNA synthetases	
VITAMIN-HORMONE RELATED		
Pernicious anemia	Anti-intrinsic factor	Etiology uncertain, vitamin B_{12} rendered physiologically unavailable
Hashimoto's disease	Antithyroglobulin common	Etiology uncertain
Insulin-dependent diabetes mellitus	Anti–beta cells of pancreas	Insulin production damaged

disease has been followed by only myasthenia gravis as a second receptor-based condition. Myelin basic protein has been identified as the critical antigen in multiple sclerosis and autoimmune variants of encephalomyelitis. Enzyme antigens are central to Reiter's syndrome, SLE, and related rheumatoid diseases.

The immunologic diagnosis of autoimmune conditions often depends on the identification of self-reactive antibodies either present in plasma or deposited in tissue. Alterations in the behavior of T cells are also a useful characteristic. Among the former group, the post-streptococcal diseases, SLE, rheumatoid arthritis, and myasthenia gravis can be listed. In these instances, complement levels may also be affected. Irregularities in T cells are noted in SLE, multiple sclerosis, and the autoimmune encephalitides. In many diseases, aberrations in both T cells and immunoglobulins have been recognized.

Therapy of autoimmune diseases has relied heavily in the past on immunosuppression, steroids, and plasmapheresis. Evidence that interleukins, such as tumor necrosis factor alpha (TNF-α), are involved in these diseases has opened a new therapeutic vista by means of passive administration of antisera. Injections of soluble antigen fragments have also been used to shield the target antigen from autoimmune effector molecules and cells.

Key Words and Phrases

Only the key words, phrases, and abbreviations appropriate to this chapter are included here.

Ankylosing spondylitis
Antigen mimicry
Antireceptor
Autoimmune hemolytic anemia
Autoimmune thrombocytopenic purpura
Bullous pemphigoid
Class I MHC genes and proteins
Class II MHC genes and proteins
Cross-reacting antigen
Dermatitis herpetiformis
Diabetes mellitus
Gm determinant
Graves' disease
Hashimoto's disease
Heat shock protein
Idiopathic thrombocytopenic purpura
Immune complex glomerulonephritis
Insulin-dependent diabetes mellitus
Multiple sclerosis
Myasthenia gravis
Neoantigen
Pemphigus vulgaris
Pernicious anemia
Polydermatositis
Post-streptococcal glomerulonephritis
Post-streptococcal rheumatic fever
Primary biliary cirrhosis
Relative risk
Rheumatic fever
Rheumatoid arthritis
Rheumatoid factor
Ribozyme
Sjögren's syndrome
Stress protein
Sympathetic ophthalmia
Systemic lupus erythematosus

Abbreviations

DP, DQ, DR	RA
FANA	RF
HLA-D region	RR
IDDM	SLE
LATS	snRNP
MBP	TNF-α
M protein	

Information Sources

Books

Bach, J.F., editor: Monoclonal antibodies and peptide therapy in autoimmune diseases, Marcel Dekker, Inc., 1993, New York.

Baillardie, F.W., editor: Autoimmunity in nephritis, Harwood Academic Publishers, 1992, Chur, Switzerland.

Bigazzi, P.E., and Reichlin, M., editors: Systemic autoimmunity, Marcel Dekker, Inc., 1991, New York.

Bigazzi, P.E., Wick, W., and Wicher, K., editors: Organ-specific autoimmunity, Marcel Dekker, Inc., 1990, New York.

Calvin, R.B., Bhan, A.K., and McCluskey, R.T. editors: Diagnostic immunopathology, Raven Press, Inc., 1988, New York.

Cruse, J.M., and Lewis, R.E., editors: Therapy of autoimmune diseases, S. Karger Publishers, Inc., 1989, Farmington, CT.

Eisenbarth, G.S.: Immunotherapy of diabetes and selected autoimmune diseases, CRC Press, Inc., 1989, Boca Raton.

Farid, N.R., editor: Immunogenetics of autoimmune disease, CRC Press, Inc., 1990, Boca Raton.

Farid, N.R., and Bona, C.A., editors: The molecular aspects of autoimmunity, Academic Press, Inc., 1990, San Diego.

Friedlaender, M.H.: Allergy and immunology of the eye, edition 2, Raven Press, Inc., 1992, New York.

Furst, D.E., and Weinblatt, M.E., editors: Immunomodulators in the rheumatic diseases, Marcel Dekker, Inc., 1990, New York.

Krawitt, E.L., and Wiesner, R.H., editors: Autoimmune liver disease, Raven Press, Inc., 1991, New York.

Oliveira, D.B.G.: Immunological aspects of renal disease, Cambridge University Press, 1992, Cambridge.

Ollier, W., and Symmons, D.P.M.: Autoimmunity, Bios Scientific Publishers, 1992, Oxford.

Pusey, C.D., editor: Immunology of renal disease, Kluwer Academic Publishers, 1991, Hingham, MA.

Samter, M., et al., editors: Immunological diseases, edition 4, Little, Brown and Co., 1988, Boston.

Talal, N., editor: Molecular autoimmunity, Academic Press, Inc., 1991, San Diego.

Voss, E.W., Jr., editor: Anti-DNA antibodies in SLE, CRC Press, Inc., 1987, Boca Raton.

Waksman, B.H., editor: Immunologic mechanisms in neurologic and psychiatric disease, Raven Press, Inc., 1990, New York.

Weetman, A.P.: Autoimmune endocrine disease, Cambridge University Press, 1991, Cambridge.

Reviews

Bernard, C.C.A., and de Rosbo, N.K.: Multiple sclerosis: an autoimmune disease of multifactorial etiology, Curr. Opin. Immunol. **4:**760, 1992.

Brostoff, S.W., and Howell, M.D.: T cell receptors, immunoregulation, and autoimmunity, Clin. Immunol. Immunopathol. **62:**1, 1992.

Charreire, J.: Immune mechanisms in autoimmune thyroiditis, Adv. Immunol. **46:**263, 1989.

Cohen, I.R.: Autoimmunity to chaperonins in the pathogenesis of arthritis and diabetes, Annu. Rev. Immunol. **9:**567, 1991.

Hansen, J.A., and Nelson, J.L.: Autoimmune diseases and HLA, Crit. Rev. Immunol. **10:**307, 1991.

Harley, J.B., and Scofield, R.H.: Systemic lupus erythematosus: RNA-protein autoantigens, models of disease heterogeneity, and theories of etiology, J. Clin. Immunol. **11:**297, 1991.

Kroemer, G., and Martínez, A.C.: Cytokines and autoimmune disease, Clin. Immunol. Immunopathol. **61:**275, 1991.

Kroemer, G., et al.: Interleukin-2, autotolerance and autoimmunity, Adv. Immunol. **50:**147, 1991.

Liblau, R.S., and Bach, J.-F.: Selective IgA deficiency and autoimmunity, Int. Arch. Allergy Immunol. **99:**16, 1992.

Linton, D.M., and Philcox, D.: Myasthenia gravis, D. M., **36:**595, 1990.

Martin, R., McFarland, H.F., and McFarlin, D.E.: Immunologic aspects of demyelinating diseases, Annu. Rev. Immunol. **10:**153, 1992.

Mason, D., and Fowell, D.: T-cell subsets in autoimmunity, Curr. Opin. Immunol. **4:**728, 1992.

Nepom, G.T., and Erlich, H.: MHC class-II molecules and autoimmunity, Annu. Rev. Immunol. **9:**493, 1991.

Steinman, L.: The development of rational strategies for selective immunotherapy against autoimmune demyelinating disease, Adv. Immunol. **49:**357, 1991.

Stollerman, G.H.: Rheumatogenic streptococci and autoimmunity, Clin. Immunol. Immunopathol. **61:**131, 1991.

Wilson, K., and Eisenbarth, G.S.: Immunopathogenesis and immunotherapy of type I diabetes, Annu. Rev. Med. **41:**497, 1990.

Wordsworth, P.: Rheumatoid arthritis, Curr. Opin. Immunol. **4:**766, 1992.

Case 1 A Different Ball Game

Greg, a 14-year-old schoolboy, was looking forward to high school and a chance to play on the interscholastic basketball team. Basketball was the only sport that Greg enjoyed, and he intended to work hard on his game before entering high school that September.

During Greg's pickup ball games during the early part of the summer, he seemed to fatigue earlier than most of his friends. Usually it was Greg who called for a break to get a drink of water. Despite his unusual perspiration, Greg also found a need for frequent visits to the gym restrooms to relieve his full bladder. Even at home in the evenings he noticed the frequent need to urinate.

These things didn't prevent him from attending Coach Tamaro's basketball camp later that summer at the university. When he arrived home 2 weeks later and received a welcome kiss from his mother, she noted that Greg's breath smelled odd, almost like ether or alcohol. After she questioned Greg about this, he told her about his other complaints of thirst, urination, and fatigue, and she arranged a visit to their family physician.

Questions

1. The physician asked Greg if he had any viral diseases in the past few months. Why?
2. What immunologic assays would you select to assist in the diagnosis of this disease?
3. At what level are T cells and immunoglobulins involved in Greg's illness?
4. Which MHC genes are associated with this disease?
5. What is its relative risk?
6. What MHC genes are negatively associated with this disease?
7. What is/are the principal antigen(s) involved here?
8. Describe the immunologic variants of this disease and their major immunologic findings.

Student Questions

Case 2 A Nervous Breakdown

Raymond F., a 56-year-old executive for a leading Midwest trucking firm, gave the following medical history. Five years earlier, when advised by his family physician that he was seriously overweight, Raymond restricted his diet and began a regular morning jogging routine. After 2 weeks, however, he developed a peculiar sensory disturbance (a feeling of numbness) in the soles of his feet that radiated into his lower legs. He temporarily halted his exercise routine for 2 or 3 weeks, and his feet began to feel much better. Rather than risk a further recurrence of his foot and leg condition, he switched to swimming. This seemed to be more satisfactory. He deliberately swam slowly with little leg kick to minimize stress on his feet, legs, and ankles.

During the past 6 months, however, he developed a noticeable weakness in his legs, causing him to take the elevator, even though his office was only on the second floor. He had recently fallen twice while walking in his home. As a result of this, he had begun to use a cane the last few weeks.

On physical examination, Raymond was moderately obese and in outward good health. Most systems appeared normal. The neurologic examination was revealing, however. Bilateral clonus of both ankles and bilateral Babinski's signs were noted. A computed tomography brain scan was unrevealing. In the apparent absence of a central nervous system (CNS) malignancy, the physician requested a series of tests from the immunology laboratory to assist him in the diagnosis of this neurologic abnormality.

Questions

1. Raymond's spinal fluid IgG was elevated and demonstrated oligoclonality. Explain the meaning of an oligoclonal IgG.
2. What is the importance of the finding that Raymond's HLA types were A3, B7, and D42.
3. Cytologic studies of spinal fluid revealed an abnormal CD4/CD8 T cell ratio. Explain.
4. Peripheral blood $CD8^+$ T cell counts were low. Explain.
5. Traces of myelin basic protein were found in the cerebrospinal fluid. Discuss myelin basic protein and its relationship to autoimmune disease.
6. Is the presence of myelin basic protein in cerebrospinal fluid incompatible with postinfectious encephalitis, Sjögren's syndrome, Lyme disease, or other CNS disease, including HIV infection?
7. Copolymer 1 was selected as a therapeutic. Discuss.
8. Adrenocorticotropic hormone was included in the therapy. Is this advisable in immune disorders of the CNS?

Student Questions

Case 3 The Sun God's Revenge

Kim said it was all Tom's fault. She had resisted Tom's efforts to arrange a spring-break ski trip all fall, only to give in at Christmas time. Now Tom was sorry he had pressured her into this.

After only 3 days on the slopes, Kim developed a rash across her cheeks and nose. She was sure it wasn't sunburn because she had used sunscreen faithfully, several times a day in fact. Moreover, she had a little pain in her wrists and fingers, which like her knees and ankles seemed slightly swollen. Kim skipped the next day's skiing because of her painful finger and wrist joints, which became heavily swollen. Later that day she noticed that she had a slight fever and a general feeling of tiredness, but what bothered her most was her blood-tinged urine.

When Tom came in for lunch and learned of this, he hurried Kim to a hospital in a nearby city, where she was examined. The physical findings were as described. Her temperature was slightly elevated, but her other vital signs were in the normal range. Urinalysis confirmed her hematuria and identified a proteinuria as well. Her hematocrit was low.

Questions

1. What immune diseases are compatible with the results of the urinalysis?
2. Which of these would be associated with a depressed hematocrit?
3. What is the immunologic basis of elevated protein levels in urine?
4. The attending physician recommended a fluorescent antinuclear antibody (ANA) test. Explain this procedure and its potential results.
5. What is/are the significant antigen(s) involved in positive fluorescent ANA tests?
6. Kim's serum was positive in tests for rheumatoid factor, yet she does not have rheumatoid arthritis. Explain.
7. What would the immunologic findings be of a kidney biopsy?

8. Explain the probable result of serum complement assays in this case.
9. What would you recommend for therapy?
10. What is the prospect that Kim's children will be affected by this same disease?

Student Questions

Case 4 This Has to "Bloody Well" Stop

Elaine T., a 32-year-old housewife, had a family history of neuroses. Her mother had been institutionalized for a disorder that resembled manic depression but had other characteristics that defied diagnosis. Elaine's father was a victim of Alzheimer's disease at the relatively young age of 55. Elaine herself had experienced several months of depression following the delivery of her only child. Although Elaine's husband thought his wife had recovered from this postpartum depression, it was clear she never experienced the joy of motherhood, had occasions of wild enthusiasm ("Let's learn Thai and move to Bangkok"), and appeared to be entering the same neurotic state as her mother. This prompted a psychological-psychiatric examination, after which Elaine was placed on medication with lithium and a tranquilizer.

Six months into therapy, Elaine began to experience gingival bleeding when she brushed her teeth. Her next menstrual period became prolonged but finally stopped after 8 days. During this time, small petechiae and a few larger hemorrhagic spots appeared on her abdomen. Her psychiatrist referred her to a colleague in internal medicine. The latter promptly ordered a platelet count and blood clotting studies. He in turn consulted with Elaine's psychiatrist about her medication.

Questions

1. Elaine's platelet count was 28,000/mm^3. Discuss this in relationship to her probable diagnosis.
2. Why or how did Elaine's illness manifest itself at this time?
3. What drugs or classes of drugs are associated with the type of illness Elaine developed?

4. What host antigens are typically involved in this disease?
5. What class(es) of immunoglobulins is/are associated with this disease?
6. Are complement levels affected in this illness?
7. What immune variants of this disease are recognized?
8. Would Coombs' tests be positive in this disease?
9. How would a change in Elaine's medication resolve her disease?
10. Does this condition have an allo-immune counterpart?

Student Questions

Case 5 The Skin Game

Ben H., a Vietnam veteran 44 years of age, was referred to the dermatology clinic of the regional VA hospital by a physician in rural South Dakota. Papulovesicular lesions on both of Ben's elbows and knees had not responded to topical corticosteroid therapy. These vesicles would dry, crust over, and be followed by a renewed cluster of vesicles. This had gone on for nearly 2 months. During his service in Vietnam, Ben had several skin diseases—athlete's foot, an ear infection, and other fungal infections—but none of them was like this.

The VA physician discounted the common vesicular skin diseases of viral etiology and thought he was dealing with one of the rare autoimmune diseases of the skin. He consulted his reference sources to determine which tests to order. He then requested a skin biopsy, ordered determinations of the serum immunoglobulin and complement levels, and MHC class I and class II determinations.

Questions

1. What immunologic assays would be performed on the tissue from the skin biopsy?
2. Assuming that some immunoglobulins are found in the skin, how does their distribution affect the diagnosis?
3. Again, on the assumption that immunoglobulins are found in the skin, how does identification of immunoglobulin class influence the diagnosis?

4. How do these immunoglobulins reach the skin—as free molecules or immune complexes? Explain.
5. In some autoimmune conditions, IgA and complement are deposited together in the skin, yet IgA doesn't "fix" complement. Explain.
6. Which complement components are most frequently found in autoimmune skin disease?
7. What is the quantitative relationship of serum immunoglobulins to those deposited in the skin?
8. What antigens are incriminated in autoimmune skin diseases?
9. What HLA class I and II relationships exist with autoimmune skin disease?
10. What would be the immunologic findings if this were a variant of discoid systemic lupus erythematosus?
11. List the autoimmune skin diseases.

Student Questions

Case 6 That's How the Ball Bounces

A 17-year-old high school athlete, Brian R., developed a severe sore throat during the Christmas–New Year's basketball tournament. He never mentioned this to his coach or family because he wanted to continue playing. He took no medication—only a few flavored throat lozenges and an occasional aspirin. By the time classes began, he was feeling perfectly well again.

Just as the state district tournament began in February, Brian noticed a soreness in his ankles but attributed it to the stress of practice and the conference tournament play. His team won both the conference and district competitions and progressed to the regionals the next week. In the first game of this tournament, Brian developed a stiff, sore right knee that became swollen and red. His ankles were also painful and swollen at this time.

In consult with the family physican, Brian was unable to recall any injury to his ankles or knees. His arm joints were not affected; neither were his wrist joints. All physical and vital signs were normal.

Questions

1. What factors suggest this is a case of rheumatoid arthritis (RA)?
2. What factors suggest this is a case of rheumatic fever (RF)?
3. What serologic tests are useful in the diagnosis of RA? Describe.
4. What serologic tests are useful in the diagnosis of RF? Describe.
5. What immunologic events in the joint space are associated with RA?
6. What other autoimmune diseases are related to RF?
7. Describe the antigens involved in the post-streptococcal diseases.
8. Describe post-streptococcal glomerulonephritis from the perspective of immunology.
9. Describe the role of neutrophils in inflammation of the glomerular basement membrane.

Student Questions

Review Questions

1. Rheumatoid factor(s)
   - A. Definitely causes rheumatoid arthritis
   - B. Is most frequently an IgM that reacts with IgG
   - C. In serum are a specific diagnostic of rheumatoid arthritis
   - D. Fail to react with Gm determinants with only rare exceptions
   - E. Are cross-reactive with group A streptococcal antigens

2. Which of the following is considered an antireceptor autoimmune disease?
   - A. Multiple sclerosis
   - B. Graves' disease
   - C. Type 1 (insulin-dependent) diabetes mellitus
   - D. Hashimoto's disease
   - E. Rheumatic fever

3. The joint presence of IgA and C3b in deposits seen in certain skin diseases

A. Proves that IgA can activate the complement system
B. Suggests that complement activation has occurred by the alternate pathway
C. Indicates that complement fixing IgG or IgM must also be in these deposits
D. Means that the patients must be hypocomplementemic
E. Proves the cell lysis seen in the skin lesions is due to complement activation

4. The immunologic target in multiple sclerosis is

A. The acetycholinesterase inhibitor
B. Acetylcholinesterase
C. Myelin basic protein
D. The T_S cell, destroyed or inhibited by an autoantibody
E. An RNA polymerase

5. Which of the following autoimmune diseases is **least** associated with an autoreactive antibody?

A. Postinfectious encephalomyelitis
B. Multiple sclerosis
C. Bullous pemphigoid
D. Systemic lupus erythematosus
E. Rheumatic fever

6. Autoantibody directed against enzymes has been reported for which of the following pairs?

A. Hashimoto's and Graves' disease
B. Rheumatic fever and post-streptococcal glomerulonephritis
C. Myasthenia gravis and multiple sclerosis
D. Pemphigus vulgaris and bullous pemphigoid
E. Systemic lupus erythematosus and Sjögren's syndrome

7. Insulin-dependent diabetes mellitus appears to be closely associated with

A. Antibody to insulin
B. Antibody to the insulin receptor
C. Anti-islet cell antibodies
D. Anti-Langerhans' cells
E. The same etiology as for type I diabetes

8. In reference to a specific disease, a **relative risk** factor of 90 means that

A. 90% of the population will develop the disease
B. 90% of the population will **not** develop the disease
C. 90% of the people who develop the disease will have a certain MHC antigen on their cells
D. 10% of the patient's with the disease will have a certain MHC antigen on their cells
E. The MHC antigen referred to in the calculation cross reacts with the critical antigen in the disease.

9. The genetic relationship of an autoimmune disease is most closely related to which genes?

A. MHC class II genes
B. MHC class III genes
C. HLA-B genes
D. MHC class I genes
E. HLA-A genes

10. A peculiar restriction in the selection of light chain immunoglobulin genes has been noted in

A. Hashimoto's disease
B. Thrombocytopenic purpura
C. Autoimmune glomerulonephritis
D. Rheumatoid arthritis
E. Pernicious anemia

17 Allergy

The allergies (hypersensitivities) are conditions created by an undesired immune response to extrinsic antigens or haptens, the latter usually creating new epitopes by their reaction with host macromolecules. The anaphylactic or type I allergies are those that depend on the reaction of antigen with its specific IgE bound to the surface of mast cells and basophils (Table 17-1). The degranulative release of vasoactive products, particularly histamine and leukotrienes C, D, and E, from these cells is responsible for the pulmonary vasoconstriction, smooth muscle contraction, and edema so characteristic of this type of allergy. Other mast cell products, platelet activating factor, eosinophil chemotactic factors, and prostacyclins, plus bradykinin and related compounds freed from plasma proteins contribute to the symptomatology of the anaphylactic allergies.

The anaphylactic reaction, especially if associated with injected antigens or haptens, which are quickly dispersed through the blood, may terminate fatally. This is less apt to be the result of food allergies or inhalant allergies, but even here fatal anaphylactic reactions may occur. Consequently, the diagnosis, prevention, and treatment of this form of allergy are very important.

The rapid appearance and spread of edema and erythema following the intradermal injection of a dilute preparation of a substance to which a person is allergic is a relatively inexpensive method to identify an IgE-based allergy. Titration of the total amount of IgE in a patient's serum may suggest that an allergy exists, even though this does not identify the offending allergens. Alternatively, serologic tests of the

Table 17-1. Major features of the hypersensitivities

	Type I	Type II	Type III	Type VI
Synonym	Anaphylactic	Cytotoxic	Immune complex	Delayed type
Immunoglobulin	IgE	IgG, IgM, and other	IgG, IgM, and other	None
Target cells	Mast cells and basophils	Erthrocytes, leukocytes, etc.	Varies	Varies
Mediators	Histamine, leukotrienes, etc.	Complement	Complement and granulocytes	T_{H1} cells, macrophages, Il-1, TNF-α
Examples	Hay fever, food allergy, penicillin allergy	Transfusion reactions	Hypersensitivity pneumonitis	Poison ivy, tuberculin reaction
Treatment	Antihistamines, catecholamines	None	Corticosteroids	Corticosteroids

person's serum with a panel of suspected allergens can identify the antigen specificity of this IgE. Ideally, the highly sensitive ELISA or radioimmunoassay (RIA) methods are used in these assays (RIST and RAST).

Treatment of the type I allergies with adrenergic drugs has two major advantages over the use of antihistamines. The first is a reversal of the effects of mast cell mediators on smooth muscle, and the second is an actual stabilization of mast cells. Antihistamines only block histamine receptors on mast cells and cannot reverse an earlier effect of histamine on smooth muscle. Other drugs are also in use to treat or prevent anaphylactic-type reactions.

Antigen-specific hyposensitization developed through the injection of the allergen is an effective method used to prevent further reactions. The success of this procedure is correlated with the production of IgG blocking antibody, an antibody in blood that intercepts circulating antigen before it reaches the IgE that is bound to mast cells in tissue.

Cytotoxic (type II) allergic reactions depend on antibodies, particularly isotypes G and M, that react with cellular antigens. In the presence of complement, this may lyse the target cell. Mismatched transfusion of erythrocytes into recipients who have preformed antibody to erythrocyte surface antigens is one example of a type II allergy. Maternal antibodies that pass the placenta and enter the fetal circulation to provoke hemolytic disease of the newborn is a second example. Such conditions are easily prevented, the former by careful blood grouping, and the latter by the administration of anti-RhD serum to the Rh-negative mother whenever she delivers or aborts an RhD-positive child.

Immune complex (type III) allergy develops when soluble complexes of antigen and antibody, frequently with components of the complement system, deposit on tissue surfaces. When blockade of the vascular bed occurs, it may be severe enough to cause local tissue necrosis (the Arthus phenomenon). Hypersensitivity pneumonitis, also known as extrinsic allergic pneumonitis, immune complex pneumonitis, or by other more specific terms (e.g., farmer's lung, pigeon-breeder's lung, mushroom worker's lung), occurs when the aveolar blood vessels are occluded. Air heavily laden with antigen is inhaled, absorbed, and reaches and precipitates with antibody in the circular system of the lung to form multiple, minute Arthus reactions.

Inflammation of the joints and edema are characteristic of serum sickness, another type III allergy. Serum therapy in transplant patients who receive equine antisera against human T cells as an immunosuppressant often causes serum sickness. Although IgG and IgM dominate these reactions, IgE may participate in its early edematous phase.

Delayed-type hypersensitivity, the type IV or cell-mediated hypersensitivity, is a T cell–based reaction that does not involve immunoglobulins. Individuals sensitized by prior dermal contact to certain chemicals will develop a thickened, erythematous rash at the point of contact that is maximal in intensity at 48 hours on recontact with the chemical. After an early infiltration of granulocytes into the skin, these cells give way to an influx of mononuclear cells. The latter release interleukin-1 (IL-1) and tumor necrosis factor alpha (TNF-α), which are important contributors to poison ivy, poison oak reactions, and other forms of contact dermatitis.

Delayed-type hypersensitivity reactions in the skin following the injection of products of infectious organisms, such as in the tuberculin reactions, constitute a second form of type IV allergy.

Key Words and Phrases

Certain items in this vocabulary may be familiar to you from your study of the earlier chapters.

ABO system
Adrenergic drug
Anaphylactoid reaction
Anaphylatoxin
Anaphylaxis
Antihistamine
Arthus reaction
Asthma
Atopy
Basophil
Blocking antibody
Bradykinin
Catecholamine
Cell-mediated hypersensitivity
Compatibility test
Contact dermatitis
Coombs' tests
Crossmatch
Cytotoxic hypersensitivity
Delayed-type hypersensitivity
Desensitization
Eosinophil
Eosinophil chemotactic factors of anaphylaxis
Fc_ε receptors
Food allergy
Hemolytic disease of the newborn
Histamine
Hypersensitivity pneumonitis
Hyposensitization
Immune complex hypersensitivity
Immune complex pneumonitis
Immunoglobulin E
Late phase reaction
Leukotrienes
Mast cells
Nonseasonal allergy
Platelet activating factor
Prausnitz-Küstner test
RAST test
Respiratory allergy
Rh system
RIST test
Seasonal allergy
Serum sickness

Information Sources

Books

Baldo, B.A., editor: Molecular approaches to the study of allergens, S. Karger Publishers, Inc., 1990, Farmington, CT.

Chadwick, D., Evered, D., and Whelan, J., editors: IgE, mast cells and the allergic response, John Wiley & Sons, Ltd., 1989, Chichester.

Daniele, R.P.: Immunology and immunologic diseases of the lung, Year Book Medical Publishers, 1988, Chicago.

Fireman, P., and Slavin, R.G.: Atlas of allergies, Raven Press, Inc., 1991, New York.

Jordan, R.E., editor: Immunologic diseases of the skin, Appleton and Lange, 1991, Norwalk, CT.

Kaliner, M.A., Barnes, P.J., and Persson, C.G.A., editors: Asthma: its pathology and treatment, Marcel Dekker, Inc., 1991, New York.

Kaliner, M.A., and Metcalf, D.D., editors: The mast cell in health and disease, Marcel Dekker, Inc., 1992, New York.

Korenblat, P.E., and Wedner, H.J., editors: Allergy: theory and practice, edition 2, W.B. Saunders Co., 1992, Philadelphia.

Metcalfe, D., Sampson, H.A., and Simon, R.A., editors: Food allergy: adverse reactions to foods and food additives, Blackwell Scientific Publications, 1991, Boston.

Middleton, E., Jr., et al., editors: Allergy, principles and practice, edition 3, C.V. Mosby, 1988, St. Louis.

Mueller, U.R.: Insect sting allergy, VCH Publishers, 1990, New York.

Patterson, R., et al., editors: Allergic diseases: diagnosis and treatment, edition 4, J.B., Lippincott Co., 1993, Philadelphia.

Samter, M., et al., editors: Immunologic diseases, edition 4, Little, Brown and Co., 1988, Boston.

Sorg, C.: Cytokines regulating the allergic response, S. Karger AG, 1989, Basel.

Spry, C.J.F.: Eosinophils: a comprehensive review and guide to the scientific and medical literature, Oxford University Press, 1988, Oxford.

Reviews

Adams, R.M.: Recent advances in contact dermatitis, Ann. Allergy **67**:552, 1991.

Arm, J.P., and Lee, T.H.: The pathobiology of bronchial asthma, Adv. Immunol. **51**:323, 1992.

Bochner, B.S., and Lichtenstein, L.M.: Anaphylaxis, N. Engl. J. Med. **324**:1785, 1991.

Chandra, R.K., et al.: Strategies for the prevention of food associated atopic disease, Adv. Exp. Biol. Med. **310**:391, 1991.

deVries, J.-E., et al.: Regulation of IgE synthesis by cytokines, Curr. Opin. Immunol. **3**:851, 1991.

George, R.B., and Owens, M.W.: Bronchial asthma, D. M. **37**:142, 1991.

Kaplan, A.P., et al.: Histamine releasing factors and cytokine-dependent activation of basophils and mast cells, Adv. Immunol. **50**:237, 1991.
Larsen, G.L.: Asthma in children, N. Engl. J. Med. **326**:1540, 1992.
Lieberman, P.: Anaphylactoid reactions to radiocontrast material, Ann. Allergy **67**:91, 1991.
Platts-Mills, T.A.: Atopic allergy: asthma and atopic dermatitis, Curr. Opin. Immunol. **3**:873, 1991.
Ravetch, J.V., and Kinet, J.-P.: Fc receptors, Annu. Rev. Immunol. **9**:457, 1991.
Sharma, O.P.: Hypersensitivity pneumonitis, D. M. **37**:415, 1991.
Weller, P.F.: Roles of eosinophils in allergy, Curr. Opin. Immunol. **4**:782, 1992.
Yunginger, J.W.: Anaphylaxis, Ann. Allergy **69**:87, 1992.

Case 1 An Itch More than Skin Deep

Ronald S., a 36-year-old man, had undergone chronic hemodialysis for the past 3 years. During the past 4 months, Ronald began to experience severe itching and swelling near the site where the arteriovenous shunt was located on his arm. This shunt is plastic at its ends but has a rubber connecting tube in its center. This reaction normally began only a few minutes after connecting the shunt.

Ronald's most recent experience included symptoms more severe than minor itching and edema. This time a tightness in his chest, shortness of breath, and a pounding in his head occurred—symptoms that prompted Ronald's dialysis team to search for the cause of the reaction.

The dialysis team knew that the plastic portion of the dialysis unit was sterilized in formaldehyde by the dialysis team technicians. This was extensively flushed with sterile saline before use. The rubber connecting tube was purchased as a unit sterilized in ethylene oxide gas by the manufacturer. This section of the shunt was discarded after each use, and a new rubber connection was used to join to the plastic unit. The patient's skin was cleansed with soap and then isopropyl alcohol prior to insertion of the shunt. Heparin was injected to minimize blood clotting during the process.

Questions

1. What type of allergic reaction was Ronald experiencing—type I, II, etc.?
2. Explain the sequence of immunologic events that led to the itching and edema.
3. How would you determine if the formaldehyde, ethylene oxide, heparin, and so on was the incitant allergen?
4. Describe the immunoglobulin(s) involved in Ronald's allergy.
5. Discuss the Fc receptors for immunoglobulins.
6. Could this be an anaphylactoid reaction?
7. What could one learn from RIST and RAST tests of Ronald's serum?
8. Describe the steps of the RIST and RAST assays.
9. Is this a type of allergy where desensitization would be attempted?

10. What drugs would you advise for Ronald's treatment if he entered into this type of reaction again?

Student Questions

Case 2 Do You Dig It?

Howard M., a 68-year-old retired professor of plant pathology, had purchased kits for raising mushrooms for the past 3 years since his retirement. These kits consisted of a wooden box containing compost that had been seeded with mushroom spores. When kept moist, the spores germinate and produce edible mushrooms. This year Howard expanded his hobby and had several kits in different stages of production in a small, closed room in his basement.

After harvesting a few mushrooms one day, Howard developed a dry cough, and a few hours later had a definite shortness of breath. He also felt like he had a slight fever, but the next morning he felt perfectly normal again. However, a week later after working with his mushroom cultures for the first time since his reaction, Howard once again experienced a dry cough, dyspnea, fever, and chills. The symptoms were most noticeable about 6 hours after working with his cultures. Uncertain as to the cause of this reaction and the risk of future reactions, Howard consulted his physician.

Questions

1. Howard had no reaction after eating raw or cooked mushrooms. Explain.
2. How do you classify this type of allergy—type I, II, etc.? Explain its immunologic basis.
3. What, if any, is the role of immunoglobulins in this allergy?
4. What, if any, is the role of complement in this allergy?
5. If the offending allergen were injected into Howard's skin, what would occur?
6. How would an antihistamine affect this reaction?
7. How are granulocytes involved in this allergic reaction?
8. Is Howard's blood safe to use in blood transfusions? Explain.

9. What antigens contribute to the various forms of this type of allergic reaction?
10. Is desensitization a logical approach to reducing Howard's allergic sensitivity?

Student Questions

Case 3 Another Way Montezuma Got Revenge

Janet B. often accompanied her dentist husband to the rural parts of Mexico where a team of his dentist friends made an annual expedition for voluntary dental care of the economically underprivileged. On one earlier occasion, Janet had a severe bout of "Montezuma's revenge" that kept her bedfast for 2 days and pretty well ruined her trip. For the past 2 years, Janet had purchased an over-the-counter preparation in Mexico that contained trimethoprim-sulfamethoxazole as a prophylactic against diarrhea.

Unfortunately, after only 3 days in Mexico on this last trip, Janet developed a severe stomatitis. Numerous vesicles appeared on her inner cheeks, under and on her tongue, and on the roof of her mouth. These were very painful and made it next to impossible for her to eat or speak. After 3 days, during which she survived almost solely on soup, the vesicles began to heal, and she felt much better. Janet concluded that this was an allergic reaction to some spicy Mexican dishes she had eaten during her first days on the trip and decided to avoid such food on her future trips.

The next year Janet again joined the volunteer dentists on their excursion, only to have the same problem of painful oral blisters arise. Since she had avoided local spicy foods on this trip, she decided this was not a simple food allergy.

Questions

1. How would you classify this allergy?
2. Would antibody be present in the vesicle fluid?
3. What is the evidence for and against this being a food allergy?
4. List drugs taken orally that are frequently involved in allergic reactions.
5. How would you use the Prausnitz-Küstner test to analyze Janet's allergy?

6. Except for avoidance of the allergen, how could this reaction be avoided?
7. What is your recommendation for treatment of this kind of allergic reaction?
8. What foods are most commonly associated with allergies?
9. What are the different manifestations of drug allergies?
10. What is the biochemical pathway leading to mast cell degranulation?

Student Questions

Case 4 A Complex Immune System

Lisa W. realized she had made a mistake. Not now, not even last week, but several months ago when vacationing in Brazil. There she had visited a few of the major cities but had enjoyed much more the small villages off the beaten path. Unfortunately, it was in just such a village she had her accident and was taken to a small government clinic, where she received a booster for her tetanus immunization. Although Lisa was very apprehensive about the reuse of "sterilized" platinum needles and boiled glass syringes, she knew the risk of tetanus was also very great and agreed to the booster immunization.

Nearly 2 months after this incident, after her return to the United States, Lisa developed a low-grade fever that persisted for several weeks. During that period, she often felt tired and had an unusual frequency of headaches and occasional cycles of fever and chills. Her illness was diagnosed as viral hepatitis type B. Gradually her symptoms resolved, and Lisa never experienced the jaundice and dark urine seen in some cases of viral hepatitis.

Now, months later, Lisa noted an increasing tenderness in her knee joints. Over the succeeding days she gradually developed pain in her wrists, ankles, and knees. Sometimes these joints became swollen and hot. Lisa realized it was time to see her doctor again. Her doctor asked for a urinalysis, which was returned as 3+ proteinuria, a fact that convinced him that a blood antigenemia assay would also be positive.

Questions

1. In what way is hepatitis B associated with arthralgia and proteinuria?
2. How is antigenemia defined? In what illnesses is persistent antigenemia a possibility?
3. Is antigenemia associated with the simultaneous presence of immunoglobulins? If so, which immunoglobulins? If not, why not?
4. How does antigenemia affect the complement system?
5. Don't complement receptors modulate the removal of excess antigen during an immune response? Explain.
6. Describe the complement receptors.
7. Would Lisa have a positive test for rheumatoid factor?
8. What is the role of granulocytes in Lisa's condition?
9. What serologic tests are used to diagnose hepatitis B infections?
10. What other antigens and haptens are incriminated in hypersensitivity reactions of this type?

Student Questions

Case 5 Food for Thought

Jeremy M. was 3 years old and was having a fun summer. The June visit to Grandma's had been great even if it lasted for only 2 weeks. Grandma let him help the adults harvest strawberries from her little patch even though Jeremy ate three and stepped on five for every berry he put in the pail. At home his mother plied him with homemade strawberry jam nearly every day.

At the end of July, Jeremy's mother decided to take some of her frozen strawberries from the freezer and make ice cream for Jeremy's fourth birthday party. The party was a great success—Jeremy received some really great presents, the kids' games went off successfully, and the cake and ice cream hit the spot. As the children left, Jeremy's mother noted her son had a broad erythematous border around his lips. Thinking it might be only strawberry stains around his mouth, she took him to the bathroom to wash his face. Then she saw that his lips were slightly swollen. Just then red splotches popped up on Jeremy's cheeks, and he began to scratch his abdomen. As she raised his T-shirt, Jeremy's mother saw several more of these red splotches.

Questions

1. Jeremy did not develop this reaction until approximately 8 weeks after his first consumption of strawberries. Explain.
2. Why didn't Jeremy react to the strawberry jam that he ate regularly?
3. What features of this case remind you of the original Prausnitz-Küstner case?
4. What is the P-K test? Is it needed here?
5. Would Jeremy's allergy be apparent in other regions of his digestive tract?
6. How does one explain the appearance of hives?
7. On later expressions of food allergy, hives often appear in exactly the same locations as noted earlier. How is this explained?
8. It is said that a person can "outgrow" their allergies. How can this happen?
9. It is also said that after one develops the first allergy, other allergies appear. How is this explained?
10. Describe the immunologic events that led to and became expressed in Jeremy's allergy.

Student Questions

Case 6 An Itch to Get Started

Ray and Jim had formed a close companionship based on their mutual love of fishing. Weekend outings to the trout streams in the southern part of the state were no more enjoyable to them than sitting on the riverbank trying to hook a catfish on stink bait. On this particular excursion, they were hiking into the strip pits for some early morning bass fishing. As they left the main path to find their way to their shortcut, Ray slipped on the dew-covered undergrowth and dropped his flashlight. The light kept shining as Ray started to reach into the growth to retrieve his lantern, but Jim was an instant quicker and handed the flashlight to Ray as he helped him to his feet.

Three days later Ray called Jim at his home to ask how he had enjoyed last weekend's catch. Jim replied in the affirmative but said he'd caught more than just fish. The fingers and back of his right hand had broken out in some small blisters. The entire area was heavily inflamed and swollen. The itch was intense, and the few antihistamines he had taken hadn't done much to relieve his discomfort. Ray offered his condolences and wondered how he had escaped this.

Questions

1. Are Jim's symptoms typical of a pure delayed-type hypersensitivity?
2. What cellular events led to this symptomatology?
3. Shouldn't the antihistamine minimize the itching?
4. How did Ray escape this allergy? Is there a genetic predisposition?
5. What haptenic or antigenic compounds initiate this type of allergy? Explain.
6. Does this allergic reaction differ immunologically from allergies of infection?
7. Is penicillin allergy ever of this type?
8. How should this allergy be treated?
9. Discuss desensitization to this form of allergy. Drops added to your morning orange juice have been recommended in the past.
10. Distinguish between T_{H1} and T_{H2} cells.

Student Questions

Review Questions

1. A positive skin test, such as that to *Candida albicans*
   A. Is a good indication that the humoral immune system is functional
   B. Is called a delayed type hypersensitivity or type IV allergic reaction
   C. Appears quickly, in a time frame similar to most allergic reactions to penicillin
   D. Is characterized by edema, erythema, and wheal
   E. Is best treated with an antihistamine

2. Cytotoxic allergy to a transfusion of allogenic erythrocytes is predominantly

A. A classic IgE-dependent allergy
B. Due to the presence of high titers of antibodies in the transfused plasma that react with the recipient's red cells
C. Dependent on antibodies in the recipient that react with the transfused red blood cells
D. Due to blood group I incompatibility
E. None of the above

3. Which of the following is highly dependent on a participation of the complement system?

A. Skin reaction to old tuberculin
B. Asthma
C. RIST assays
D. Anaphylactic allergy
E. Serum sickness

4. Hyposensitization (desensitization) against ragweed pollen

A. Elevates levels of IgG that are pollen specific
B. Stops the synthesis of the leukotrienes
C. Neutralizes the mast cell receptors for histamine
D. Neutralizes the smooth muscle cell receptors for histamine
E. None of the above

5. Allergic pneumonitis is

A. Seasonal in some patients but nonseasonal in others
B. Basically an Arthus reaction in the lung
C. Classified as an immune complex hypersensitivity
D. Largely due to IgG, but other antibodies may be involved
E. All of the above

6. A skin biopsy of a site where a delayed-type hypersensitivity reaction is at its maximal stage will reveal

A. Epidermal necrosis
B. Immunoglobulin and complement deposits
C. Extensive edema
D. A mononuclear cell infiltration
E. Mast cells coated with IgE

7. The RAST and RIST tests

A. Both detect IgE specific for an antigen (allergen)
B. Measure IgE by simple binding, not by precipitation, complement fixation, or other antigen-antibody cross-linking reactions
C. Are fluorescent antibody reactions
D. Measure IgE bound to mast cells
E. Can be performed only by the ELISA technique

8. A patient with severe asthma receives little relief from antihistamines because the most important contributor to the symptoms is/are

A. Leukotrienes
B. Serotonin
C. Bradykinin
D. Adrenalin
E. None of the above

9. A child stung by a bee experiences respiratory distress within minutes and falls to the ground unconscious. This reaction is mediated by

A. The direct toxic action of bee venom
B. Sensitized T cells
C. Complement binding antibodies
D. Blocking antibody
E. IgE

10. A reaction to poison ivy or poison oak is

A. Easily prevented by blocking antibody
B. A T-cell mediated reaction
C. Typical of a person's first contact with these plants
D. Due to complete antigens of the plant that induce a specific antibody response
E. Answers C and D

Answers

Chapter 2

1. B
2. C
3. C
4. E
5. D
6. D
7. A
8. E
9. C
10. E

Chapter 3

1. C
2. D
3. C
4. C
5. C
6. A
7. C
8. E
9. C
10. E
11. E
12. D
13. B
14. B
15. E

Chapter 4

1. D
2. A
3. E
4. B
5. B
6. B
7. E
8. B
9. E
10. A
11. C
12. B
13. B
14. D
15. B

Chapter 5

1. D
2. E
3. E
4. B
5. D
6. C
7. B
8. A
9. E
10. E
11. A
12. C
13. B
14. C
15. E

Chapter 6

1. B
2. C
3. C

4. A
5. E
6. C
7. B
8. D
9. E
10. B

Chapter 7

1. E
2. B
3. D
4. B
5. C
6. E
7. E
8. E
9. B
10. A

Chapter 8

1. B
2. D
3. A
4. B
5. C
6. E
7. D
8. B
9. E
10. A

Chapter 9

1. A
2. A
3. A
4. B
5. A
6. C
7. B
8. C
9. A
10. B

11. A
12. B

Chapter 10

1. B
2. E
3. B
4. B
5. B
6. B
7. E
8. D
9. A
10. C

Chapter 11

1. A
2. C
3. D
4. C
5. A
6. B
7. D
8. A
9. C
10. B

Chapter 12

1. B
2. D
3. C
4. D
5. C
6. A
7. E
8. A
9. C

Chapter 13

1. C
2. B
3. E
4. A

5. D
6. B
7. C
8. D
9. B
10. E

Chapter 14

1. D
2. D
3. C
4. A
5. B
6. E
7. C
8. E
9. A
10. C

Chapter 15

1. E
2. E
3. C
4. B
5. A
6. D
7. C
8. B
9. E
10. B

Chapter 16

1. B
2. B
3. B
4. C
5. A
6. E
7. C
8. C
9. A
10. D

Chapter 17

1. B
2. C
3. E
4. A
5. E
6. D
7. B
8. A
9. E
10. B

Index

Note: Page numbers followed by *t* indicate tabular material.